INNA VOLIA

The 30 day
KETOGENIC
DIET

Weight Loss Cleanse, Cookbook Diet.

Contents

Introduction **6**

Defining a "Keto" Diet 8

Why does a Ketogenic Diet work? 9

Introducing Ketosis 10

Symptoms of Ketosis 11

Some key techniques to enter attain optimum Ketosis 11

Some physical effects to be aware of 12

Advantages of a Ketogenic Diet 14

Does a Ketogenic Diet help to burn fat? A Scientific Study 14

How does a Keto diet contribute to the Fat burning process 18

A quick look at the allowed ingredients of Keto Diet 19

Awesome tips to help you in your Keto journey 22

Week 1 24

Week 2 38

Week 3 52

Week 4 66

Extra 2 days! 80

Chapter 1: Breakfast Recipes **85**

Turn Of the Century Caprese Salad 85

The Melodious Spring Salad 87

Great Tomatoes With Poached Up Eggs 89

Clean Ham and Apple Flatbread 92

Nice and Juicy Creamed Spinachlings 95

A Cool Salad For Early Morning 97

A Carbonara Of Pumpkins 99

Curious Flatbread and Corned Beef 101

Fancy Chicken Roulades Ala Gruyere 103

Fan Favorite Pancake 106

Old Tale's Bacon Cheddar and Chive Omelet 108

Beautiful Shrimp and Peanut Curry Dish 110

Chapter 2: Lunch Recipes **113**

Generously Given Nasi Lemak.. 113

Delicious Popper Mug Cakes Of Jalapeno............................ 115

Molten Tuna Bites.. 117

Pigs in a Blanket.. 119

Skirt Steak With Cilantro Paste 121

Smooth Cauliflower Fried Rice (For Vegetable Lovers) 123

Pulled Pork On Top Of Cornbread Waffles 125

Glorious Reversed Bacon Burger... 127

Slow and Crazy Keto Chicken Tikka Masala.......................... 129

Swift Pizza Frittata!.. 131

Chapter 3: Dinner Recipes **133**

Sandwich Of Bacon and Healthy Avocado............................ 133

Authentic Keto Compatible Sushi... 135

Bok Choy Salad With Tofu Tossed In.................................... 137

Cute Sausage And Pepper Soup 140

Cheese and Ham and Keto Stromboli................................... 142

Meatballs Of Turky! 144

A Very Low Carb Chicken Satay 146

Slow Cooker Braised Oxtails... 148

Perfectly Braised Short Ribs.. 150

Kung Pao Chicken.. 152

Terrific County Side Gravy 154

Unlimited Delight Sesame Salmon.. 156

Chapter 4: Snacks Recipes **158**

Sinking Boats Of Molten Cheese And Zucchini...................... 158

The Most Heart Touching Grand Ma's Hot Chili Soup 160

Pleasing Amaretto Cookies.. 162

The Lightning Fast Kimchi Meal 165

Feisty Chocolate Drizzled Macaroons.................................... 168

Very Healthy Spinach and Cucumber Mix.............................. 170

Fantastic Apple Cider Worth Dying For 172

Tender Soft Pizza Fat Bombs 174
Beautiful Chocolate Milk Shake With Blackberries 176
Happily Ever After Tater Tots... 178
Lovely Potato Gratin.. 180
Fried Kale Sprouts 182

Chapter 5: Desert Recipes **184**
Cheddar and Cheese Waffles To Die For............................... 184
The Mystifying McGriddle Casserole 186
Gentle Breeze Strawberry Popsicles 188
Soft and Delightful Pumpkin Fudge.. 190
A Cool Bowl of Sausage And Cheese..................................... 192
Cute and Cuddly Vanilla Cloud Muffins................................... 194
Fine Donut Muffins With Sprinkled Sugar 196
Delightful Choco And Peanut Tart... 199
A Fine Smoothie Of Blueberry Banana Bread 202
Adorable Tartlets... 204
A Very Private and Intimate Portobello Pizza 207
Egg Drop Soup Of 5 Minutes 209
Amazing Raspberry Pavlovas 211
Magical Cashew Bars (No Bake Required)............................. 213
Mesmerizing Lemon Soufflé!... 215

Conclusion.. **217**

Introduction

First and foremost, I would like to thank you for purchasing this book and supporting me in my journey.

Since you are reading this book, I am assuming that you are interested/ or have at least heard of the diet known as the "Ketogenic" diet.

If the answer to that is an astounding "Yes", then you have come to the right place!

The target audiences for my book are absolute beginners who are just trying to scratch the surface of the Ketogenic diet, but are feeling lost, due to the thousands of different information and opinions out there.

Keeping that in mind, I took the liberty of adding this very fleshed out introductory chapter before the recipes. If you are an absolute beginner, then this chapter will walk you through all of the basic fundamentals of an Ketogenic Diet.

And even if you are already experienced in the concept of an Ketogenic Diet, you can still explore this chapter as it will help you clear up any confusions that you may have.

The chapter has been carefully designed and is broken down into tiny sections to make it as convenient and accessible to you as possible.

By the end of the introductory chapter, you have a firm idea of:

- How to define a Ketogenic Diet

- A simple outline of how a Ketogenic Diet really works

- How Ketosis works

- What are the symptoms of Ketosis

- Know about some of the key techniques of attaining optimum Ketosis

- Understand the side effects of Ketosis

- Get to know the advantage of Ketosis

- Get to know how Ketogenic Diet can greatly help you lose excess weight, proved with a full fledge Scientific Study

- Know which ingredients are allowed and prohibited during a Keto journey

- Know some amazing tips to improve the efficiency of your Keto journey

- Fully understand how to prepare a 28 days meal plan, illustrated through a given example

Defining a "Keto" Diet

A Ketogenic diet is undoubtedly one of the most well-known yet misunderstood diet out there in the open field of hundreds of different diets right now. So let's start off by defining the diet itself!

In the most Laymen's of terms, a Ketogenic Diet is a form of diet that restricts your body from ingesting a large amount of carbohydrate, thereby inducing it into a state of "Ketosis".

During Ketosis, the body tends to breakdown a large amount of fat to produce energy for the body, which eventually helps to get to rid of the excess body fat and keep the body lean and healthy.

This is done thanks to the increased production of a chemical called "Ketones" that is generated in large amount in our liver whenever the body enters Ketosis.

There are multiple names through which a Ketogenic Diet is addressed. Some prefer to call it a Low Carb-High Fat Diet while others tend to call it a Low Carb High Protein Diet.

For the sake of simplicity, here we are simply going to address it by its original name, the Ketogenic Diet.

Why does a Ketogenic Diet work?

To fully understand how a Ketogenic Diet works, you must first appreciate the fact that the Glucose/Carbohydrates are the most easily convertible molecule of our body, and is the prime source of energy.

Whenever we are ingesting any form of food that has a high carbohydrate count, the body immediately starts to generate substantial amount of glucose and insulin.

Whenever the body needs a good jolt of energy, it immediately starts to breakdown a large number of carbohydrates in order to generate the required amount of energy.

Alternatively, the insulin in our body allows the glucose to easily travel around the blood stream. Since the body prefers to use Glucose as its primary source of energy, with the help of Insulin, glucose is always taken up instead of fat!

This results in your fat being stored all around your body as unwanted body mass.

Whenever you are encouraging your body to enter Ketosis through your Ketogenic Diet, you are essentially causing it ignore carbohydrates (the little that is present) in our body and opt to burn more fat in order to generate the required energy.

The amount of fat burnt largely depends on the amount of Ketones that are produced , which in turn depends on how optimally you are able to enter and hold your state of Ketosis.

Introducing Ketosis

As I mentioned earlier, the main goal of undergoing a Ketogenic Diet is to influence your body into entering a state of "Ketosis" right?

Let me walk you through the process of Ketosis in details now.

So, basically speaking "Ketosis" is, in fact, a very normal internal metabolic process which helps to keep our body supplied with enough energy to carry out day to day activities.

Essentially what happens here is that, whenever you are depriving your body of Carbohydrates, it starts to burn down fat for energy due to the shortage of Carbohydrates. During this process, a chemical called "Ketones".

Whenever you are in a completely balanced diet, your body prevents itself from burning fat and as a result, Ketones are not produced.

This also makes Ketones a significant "Marker" for you to easily assess if your body is indeed in a state of Ketosis or not.

Aside from Ketosis, other scenarios where Ketones are produced include pregnancy and after heavy exercise.

Below are signs and symptoms which you might want to keep an eye out for to ensure that you have perfectly entered into a state of Ketosis.

Symptoms of Ketosis

- Your mouth will feel dry, and you feel have increased thirst

- The number of washroom visits will increase as you might need to urinate more often.

- Your breath will have a slight "Fruity" smell to it that will resemble that of a nail polish

- Aside from those three, you will obviously get the sensation mentioned above of having a low hunger level and increased bodily energy.

Some key techniques to enter attain optimum Ketosis

By now you should be clear that the effectiveness of a Ketogenic diet depend on the level of your Ketosis your body is able to achieve.

While simply lowering down your carbohydrate intake will most definitely help you enter Ketosis, the following tips will not only help you to enhance the effectiveness of your Ketosis, but also allow your body to stay in a state of Ketosis for a longer period of time.

- Keep your daily carbohydrate intake below 20 carbs

- Keep your protein levels at around 70g per day

- Don't starve! Swallow adequate level of fat. Remember that the body is going to need fat to burn fat.

- Try to avoid snack times and stick to your breakfast, lunch and dinner meals with nothing in between.

Some physical effects to be aware of

While a Ketogenic Diet can largely be considered as a diet without any side effects, there are still some physical changes and symptoms that you should be aware of.

During a Ketogenic Diet, you are completely changing the normal food intake of your body, which causes the homeostatic system of your body to bring about some changes and produce enzymes that might easily digest the type of food that you are consuming.

During the early stages of these changes, you are prone to experiencing symptoms such as

- Dizziness

- Aggravation

- Headaches

- Keto-Flu

- Mental Fogginess

Aside from those, some symptoms which you should be aware of are:

- **Frequent desire to urinate:** Since Ketosis will cause your body to burn up more fat, the glycogen gets stored up. In this situation, your Kidneys will start to process a lot of water and excrete them, increasing your desire to urinate.

- **Hypoglycemia:** This simply means that your sugar level might lower down

- **Constipation:** This is yet another side effect experience by some which take place due to dehydration and lower salt presence in the body. But this can very easily be tackled by drinking more water

- **Increased Sugar Craving:** During the early stage of your diet, you might get a serious craving for sugar. To tackle this, simply take some extra protein and Vitamin B Complex. A good and healthy walk works good as well.

- **Diarrhea:** This is a common issue which is faced by some people during the first few days, but it resolves itself automatically after a few days.

- **Sleep problem:** This might be a result of the reduce levels of serotonin or insulin.

You should also be aware of the fact that during Ketosis, the body tends to lose a great amount of electrolytes. This "Flushing" is partly responsible for the above mentioned side effects.

However, this diuretic effect can be tackled very easily, simply by consuming a great amount of water.

Also, if possible, you should increase your salt intake as well!

Regardless, keep in mind that if you are experiencing any of the above discussed symptoms, nothing is going wrong as they are pretty normal and will eventually go away.

Advantages of a Ketogenic Diet

With the core concept out of the way, here are the main advantages of a Keto diet

- A good Keto diet will help you to lower the levels of bad cholesterol so to prevent arterial blocks from occurring

- Energy taken from burning body fat will always keep you energetic since body fat is present in abundance in our body

- The levels of LDL will decrease which will make the body less prone to suffer from Type-2 Diabetes

- You won't always feel hungry

- Ketosis helps to improve skin condition and prevent acnes or skin inflammation from taking place.

Does a Ketogenic Diet help to burn fat? A Scientific Study

Unlike many other diets, Ketogenic is not a one, which solely relies on the word of the mouth alone. In fact, there have been multiple studies all around the world that seamlessly proves the effectiveness of a Ketogenic Diet without fail. One of the more recent studies did a fantastic job of answering this question.

a team of around eight research scientists took a notion of bringing into contrast the effectiveness of an Atkins Diet (equivalent to a Keto Diet) with three other different forms of diet over a period of 12 months completely randomized control trial.

The participants of this experiment included a broad range of 311 individuals who ranged from obese people and women who had menopause. It was strictly maintained though that none of the patients had a history of any form of cardiovascular or diabetic symptoms.

An average age of 41 years was measured of the sample, following a BMI of 32 with body fat which clocked at a percentage of 40%

After establishing these basal standards, the scientists divide the whole sample into four different groups based on the type of diet they were exposed to.

- Group-1 comprised of 76 people and were instructed to consume an Ornish Diet which had just about 10% lowered down calorie in comparison to the fatty foods.

- Group 2 had 79 participants and they were asked to go through a LEARN Diet which comprised of the same 10% fewer calories, but this time it came from the saturated fats, while 55-60% of the calorie came from the carbohydrates. The psychological and physiological activities of this group were also monitored.

- Group 3 comprising of 79 people was exposed to something called the "Zone Diet" which consisting of roughly 30%, 40% and 30% distribution of calories coming from protein, carbohydrate and fats respectively.

- Group 4 had a number of 77 participants. They were treated with a diet of the low-carb "Atkins" diet.

For all of the diets, each subject was exposed to only 20 grams of carbs per day for 2-3 months. After which they were instructed to eat 50g per day for the coming 9-10 months.

The test subjects were strictly asked to maintain the specified calorie deficit and take professional support to adjust their level of diet accordingly to ensure that they are able to adhere to the specified diet while being healthy as well.

Aside from the diet routine, the researchers also invoked a nice routine of exercise and nutritional supplements to make sure that they were not losing their healthy physique.

As you can already tell by now, the whole experiment was pretty elaborate and well thought out and the conclusion, well unsurprisingly all of the diets had shown a good amount of reduction in BMI and overall weight alongside body fat percentage. But, the one that showed the greatest decline was the Atkins diet which closely resembled the diet of a Ketogenic style.

The graph up pretty much sums up the whole scenario nicely. As you can see, the decrease in BMI of the Atkins group decreases by 1.65. In comparison, it only fell by 0.92 in the LEARN group, 0.77 in the Ornish group and a disappointing 0.53 in the Zone group.

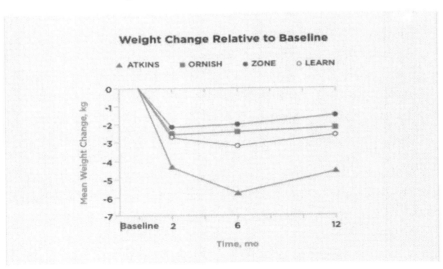

The same is seen in the bar chart below.

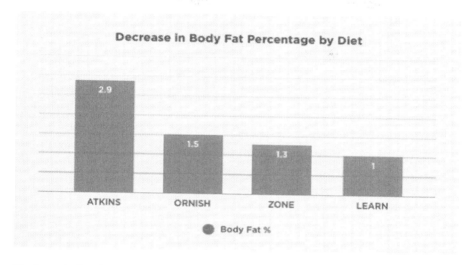

Decrease in Body Fat Percentage by Diet

But not that's not all! If you just have a look at the decline in body fat percentage that was trimmed down, the effects were more astonishing! The recorded rate decrease from the Atkins diet was at an astounding 2.9% while the others had a decline of around 1.5%, 1.3% and 1% in the Ornish, Zone, and LEARN group respectively. This even further supports the theory of the effectiveness of a low carb diet.

So, the conclusion? Yes. Through the tests done under an Atkins Diet, it can very easily be inferred that a Ketogenic Diet has the potentiality to trim down those pesky body fats and return you to the physique which you were dreaming for!

This incidentally meant that the Atkins group, which was on a diet with much decrease carb intake that the other two groups, showed significantly plausible results.

Consequently, this led to people all around the world to believe that it is indeed possible to trim down fat using a diet of Low-Carb, which is in our case, A Ketogenic Diet.

How does a Keto diet contribute to the Fat burning process

It is pretty clear now that a Ketogenic Diet does indeed help an individual to burn their excess body fat. The following are some of the ways through which Keto helps to achieve this effect

- A Ketogenic diet directly helps to increase the level of fat burnt throughout the whole day through exercise and daily activities

- A Keto Diet will cause the body to consume a significant amount of protein, consequently promoting the weight loss of the body.

- When the body is restricted from consuming Carbohydrates, the calorie intake will also lower down further contributing to weight loss.

- A process called Gluconeogenesis will kick in as well which will cause the body to burn even more fat.

- Speaking of burning fat, A Ketogenic diet will also help you to Suppress your Appetite, so you won't have to go out and eat now and then and bulk up, even more, fat.

A quick look at the allowed ingredients of Keto Diet

Fats

Go For

- Saturated Fat like coconut oil ghee
- Monosaturated Fat like olive, macadamia, almond oil
- Polyunsaturated Omega 3s as sardines
- Medium Chain Triglycerides such as fatty acid
- Lard
- Chicken Fat
- Duck Fat
- Goose Fat

Not Go For

- Refined Fats and Oil as sunflower, soybean, corn oil, etc.
- Trans Fat such as margarine

Protein

Go For

- Grass fed meat
- Harvested seafood and wild caught meat
- Free-range organic egg
- Beef
- Lamb
- Goat
- Venison
- Pastured Pork
- Poultry

Not Go For

- Factory packed animal foods and produced

Vegetable

Go For

- Leafy green vegetables
- Low carb vegetables
- Swiss chard
- Bok Choy
- Lettuce
- Chard
- Chives
- Endives
- Radicchio

Not Go For

- High starchy= high carb vegetables such as peas, potatoes, yucca, beans, legumes.

Dairy Products

Go For

- Dairy products such as yogurt, sour cream, cottage cheese, goat cheese

Not Go For

- Milk

Fruits

Go For

- In general, go for fruits that are on low carb and have more fat such as berries, avocados, etc.

Not Go For

- Try to avoid dried fruits that are high in sugar content

Drinks

Go For

- Water
- Black Coffee
- Unsweetened and Herbal Teas
- Nut Milks
- Light Beet
- Wine

Not Go For

- Drinks such as Pepsi or Coke
- High Fructose Syrup
- Nectar
- Honey
- Sodas

Sweets

Go For

- Stevia
- Xylitol
- Erythritol
- Inulin
- Monk Fruit Powder
- Cocoa Dark Chocolate

Not Go For

- Milk

Awesome tips to help you in your Keto journey

- Get yourself a good quality carb counter to keep track of your daily carb intake

- Clear out your pantry off any high-carb produce

- Restock your pantry with produces and ingredients that are compatible with your Keto diet

- Make a nice and easy to follow Diet plan (one provided)

- Remember to keep a good dose of water close to you and stay hydrated throughout the day

- Once you have decided that you are going to jump into a Ketogenic Diet, one thing which you might find interesting to follow is a technique known as "Intermittent fasting".

  This basically tells you that you should start a pre-phase of low carb diets before actually starting the diet itself, to allow your body to adjust and re-orient itself to the coming changes.

  This fasting method is comprised of two phases. Namely the Building phase (Time between first and last meal) and the cleaning phase (Time between last and first meal). Try to maintain a time period of 12 hour between the cleansing phase and 8 hours between the building phases for a start. Then keep on growing from that.

- Make sure to keep your sodium intake in check to avoid future problems during your Ketogenic journey. Easy steps may include

✓ Drinking organic broth if possible

✓ Taking a just a pinch of pink salt with you consumed meals

✓ Adding about ¼ teaspoon of pink salt to 16 ounces of water consumed

✓ Adding vegetables such as kelp to your dishes

✓ Eating up vegetables such as cucumber or celery for a more natural approach to sodium replenishment

- Try to maintain a proper exercise regime while going on your Ketogenic Diet, as it will not only help to make your Keto diet much more effective but also put a positive impact on your overall health while allowing you to maintain a more stable and prolonged state of ketosis.

A sample exercise routine may include

✓ Monday: Resistance training for upper body (20 minutes)

✓ Tuesday: Resistance training for Lower Body (20 minutes)

✓ Wednesday: Long walk of 30 minutes

✓ Thursday: Resistance training for upper body (20 minutes)

✓ Friday: Resistance training for Lower Body (20 minutes)

✓ Sat/Sun: Recreational time.

Week 1

The following is an amazing 28 days meal plan that should give you an idea of how you should prepare your own meal plan!
Keep in mind that all of the recipes used in this meal plant are available in this book.

The general guideline is to keep your daily carb intake somewhere around 30-50 carbs.

As long you are keeping your carbs in check, you can always replace these recipes with your favorite ones!

Day 1	Total Count: • Protein: 70 • Carbs: 18.83 • Fats: 103g • Calories: 1248
Breakfast	Turn Of The Century Caprese Salad • Protein: 15g • Carbs: 3.5g • Fats: 36g • Calories: 405

Snack	**Sinking Boats Of Molten Cheese And Zucchini** • Calories: 237 • Fat: 20g • Carbohydrates: 7g • Protein: 10g
Lunch	**Generously Given Nasi Lemak** • Protein: 1.4g • Carbs: 0.7g • Fats: 2.7g • Calories: 32
Dinner	**Sandwich of Bacon and Healthy Avocado** • Protein: 22g • Carbs: 4g • Fats: 28g • Calories: 361
Desert	**Cheddar and Cheese Waffles To Die For** • Protein: 6g • Carbs: 3.81g • Fats: 17g • Calories: 213

Day 2	**Total Count:** • Protein: 89 • Carbs: 33g • Fats: 168g • Calories: 1655
Breakfast	**The Melodious Spring Salad** • Carbs: 6.7g • Fats: 37.3g • Calories: 478 • Protein:: 5g
Snack	**The Most Heart Touching Grand Ma's Hot Chili Soup** • Protein: 28g • Carbs: 10.8g • Fats: 27g • Calories: 395

Lunch	**Delicious Popper Mug Cakes Of Jalapeno** • Protein: 16.5g • Carbs: 8.4g • Fats: 38g • Calories: 429
Dinner	**Authentic Keto Compatible Sushi** • Protein: 18g • Carbs: 5.7g • Fats: 25g • Calories: 353
Desert	**The Mystifying McGriddle Casserole** • Protein: 22.6g • Carbs: 2.9g • Fats: 41g • Calories: 481

Day 3	**Total Count:** • Protein: 50 • Carbs: 17g • Fats: 90g • Calories: 1036
Breakfast	**Great Tomatoes With Poached Up Eggs** • Protein: 16g • Carbs: 5g • Fats: 20g • Calories: 255
Snack	**Pleasing Amaretto Cookies** • Protein: 2.4g • Carbs: 2.5g • Fats: 7.9g • Calories: 85.7
Lunch	**Molten Tuna Bites** • Protein: 6.2g • Carbs: 2.0g • Fats: 11.8g • Calories: 134

Dinner	**Bok Choy Salad With Tofu Tossed In** • Protein: 25g • Carbs: 5.7g • Fats: 35g • Calories: 442
Desert	**Gentle Breeze Strawberry Popsicles** • Protein: 0.5g • Carbs: 2g • Fats: 16g • Calories: 150

Day 4	**Total Count:** • Protein: 70 • Carbs: 18.83 • Fats: 103g • Calories: 1248
Breakfast	**Turn Of The Century Caprese Salad** • Protein: 15g • Carbs: 3.5g • Fats: 36g • Calories: 405
Snack	**Sinking Boats Of Molten Cheese And Zucchini** • Calories: 237 • Fat: 20g • Carbohydrates: 7g • Protein: 10g
Lunch	**Generously Given Nasi Lemak** • Protein: 1.4g • Carbs: 0.7g • Fats: 2.7g • Calories: 32

Dinner	**Sandwich of Bacon and Healthy Avocado** • Protein: 22g • Carbs: 4g • Fats: 28g • Calories: 361
Desert	**Cheddar and Cheese Waffles To Die For** • Protein: 6g • Carbs: 3.81g • Fats: 17g • Calories: 213

Day 5	Total Count: • Protein: 89 • Carbs: 33g • Fats: 168g • Calories: 1655
Breakfast	**The Melodious Spring Salad** • Carbs: 6.7g • Fats: 37.3g • Calories: 478 • Protein:: 5g
Snack	**The Most Heart Touching Grand Ma's Hot Chili Soup** • Protein: 28g • Carbs: 10.8g • Fats: 27g • Calories: 395
Lunch	**Delicious Popper Mug Cakes Of Jalapeno** • Protein: 16.5g • Carbs: 8.4g • Fats: 38g • Calories: 429

Dinner	**Authentic Keto Compatible Sushi** • Protein: 18g • Carbs: 5.7g • Fats: 25g • Calories: 353
Desert	**The Mystifying McGriddle Casserole** • Protein: 22.6g • Carbs: 2.9g • Fats: 41g • Calories: 481

Day 6	**Total Count:** • Protein: 50 • Carbs: 17g • Fats: 90g • Calories: 1036
Breakfast	**Great Tomatoes With Poached Up Eggs** • Protein: 16g • Carbs: 5g • Fats: 20g • Calories: 255
Snack	**Pleasing Amaretto Cookies** • Protein: 2.4g • Carbs: 2.5g • Fats: 7.9g • Calories: 85.7
Lunch	**Molten Tuna Bites** • Protein: 6.2g • Carbs: 2.0g • Fats: 11.8g • Calories: 134

Dinner	**Bok Choy Salad With Tofu Tossed In** • Protein: 25g • Carbs: 5.7g • Fats: 35g • Calories: 442
Desert	**Gentle Breeze Strawberry Popsicles** • Protein: 0.5g • Carbs: 2g • Fats: 16g • Calories: 150

Day 7	**Total Count:** • Protein: 89 • Carbs: 33g • Fats: 168g • Calories: 1655
Breakfast	**The Melodious Spring Salad** • Carbs: 6.7g • Fats: 37.3g • Calories: 478 • Protein:: 5g
Snack	**The Most Heart Touching Grand Ma's Hot Chili Soup** • Protein: 28g • Carbs: 10.8g • Fats: 27g • Calories: 395
Lunch	**Delicious Popper Mug Cakes Of Jalapeno** • Protein: 16.5g • Carbs: 8.4g • Fats: 38g • Calories: 429

Dinner	**Authentic Keto Compatible Sushi** • Protein: 18g • Carbs: 5.7g • Fats: 25g • Calories: 353
Desert	**The Mystifying McGriddle Casserole** • Protein: 22.6g • Carbs: 2.9g • Fats: 41g • Calories: 481

Week 2

Day 1	**Total Count:** • Protein: 72 • Carbs: 20g • Fats: 58g • Calories: 1823
Breakfast	**Clean Ham and Apple Flatbread** • Protein: 16g • Carbs: 4g • Fats: 20g • Calories: 1306
Snack	**The Lightning Fast Kimchi Meal** • Protein: 27.3g • Carbs: 9.5g • Fats: 20g • Calories: 334

Lunch	**Pigs In A Blanket** • Protein: 4g • Carbs: 1g • Fats: 6g • Calories: 72
Dinner	**Cute Sausage and Pepper Soup** • Protein: 27g • Carbs: 3.8g • Fats: 2.3g • Calories: 525
Desert	**Soft and Delightful Pumpkin Fudge** • Protein: 1.2g • Carbs: 1.63g • Fats: 10g • Calories: 120

Day 2	**Total Count:** • Protein: 85 • Carbs: 23g • Fats: 89g • Calories: 1278
Breakfast	**Nice and Juicy Creamed Spinachlings** • Protein: 6g • Carbs: 4g • Fats: 13g • Calories: 157
Snack	**Feisty Chocolate Drizzled Macarrons** • Protein: 2.2g • Carbs: 2.5g • Fats: 6.8g • Calories: 76.5
Lunch	**Skirt Steak With Cilantro Paste** • Protein: 32.3g • Carbs: 2.8g • Fats: 32.5g • Calories: 432

Dinner	**Cheese and Ham Keto Stromboli** • Protein: 25g • Carbs: 9g • Fats: 21g • Calories: 305
Desert	**A Cool Bowl Of Sausage And Cheese** • Protein: 20g • Carbs: 5g • Fats: 16.7 • Calories: 308

Day 3	**Total Count:** • Protein: 88 • Carbs: 34g • Fats: 152g • Calories: 1925
Breakfast	**A Cool Salad For Early Morning** • Calories: 417 • Fat: 31g • Carbohydrates: 2.55g • Protein: 29g
Snack	**Very Healthy Spinach and Cucumber Mix** • Protein: 3g • Carbs: 7g • Fats: 33g • Calories: 335
Lunch	**Smooth Cauliflower Fried Rice** • Protein: 34g • Carbs: 19.4g • Fats: 48g • Calories: 685

Dinner	**Meatball Of Turky** • Protein: 12g • Carbs: 0.8g • Fats: 10.3g • Calories: 141
Desert	**Cute And Cuddly Vanilla Cloud Muffins** • Protein: 10g • Carbs: 5g • Fats: 30g • Calories: 347

Day 4	Total Count: • Protein: 72 • Carbs: 20g • Fats: 58g • Calories: 1823
Breakfast	**Clean Ham and Apple Flatbread** • Protein: 16g • Carbs: 4g • Fats: 20g • Calories: 1306
Snack	**The Lightning Fast Kimchi Meal** • Protein: 27.3g • Carbs: 9.5g • Fats: 20g • Calories: 334
Lunch	**Pigs In A Blanket** • Protein: 4g • Carbs: 1g • Fats: 6g • Calories: 72

Dinner	**Cute Sausage and Pepper Soup** • Protein: 27g • Carbs: 3.8g • Fats: 2.3g • Calories: 525
Desert	**Soft and Delightful Pumpkin Fudge** • Protein: 1.2g • Carbs: 1.63g • Fats: 10g • Calories: 120

Day 5	**Total Count:** • Protein: 85 • Carbs: 23g • Fats: 89g • Calories: 1278
Breakfast	**Nice and Juicy Creamed Spinachlings** • Protein: 6g • Carbs: 4g • Fats: 13g • Calories: 157
Snack	**Feisty Chocolate Drizzled Macarrons** • Protein: 2.2g • Carbs: 2.5g • Fats: 6.8g • Calories: 76.5
Lunch	**Skirt Steak With Cilantro Paste** • Protein: 32.3g • Carbs: 2.8g • Fats: 32.5g • Calories: 432

Dinner	**Cheese and Ham Keto Stromboli** • Protein: 25g • Carbs: 9g • Fats: 21g • Calories: 305
Desert	**A Cool Bowl Of Sausage And Cheese** • Protein: 20g • Carbs: 5g • Fats: 16.7 • Calories: 308

Day 6	Total Count: • Protein: 88 • Carbs: 34g • Fats: 152g • Calories: 1925
Breakfast	**A Cool Salad For Early Morning** • Calories: 417 • Fat: 31g • Carbohydrates: 2.55g • Protein: 29g
Snack	**Very Healthy Spinach and Cucumber Mix** • Protein: 3g • Carbs: 7g • Fats: 33g • Calories: 335
Lunch	**Smooth Cauliflower Fried Rice** • Protein: 34g • Carbs: 19.4g • Fats: 48g • Calories: 685

Dinner	**Meatball Of Turky** • Protein: 12g • Carbs: 0.8g • Fats: 10.3g • Calories: 141
Desert	**Cute And Cuddly Vanilla Cloud Muffins** • Protein: 10g • Carbs: 5g • Fats: 30g • Calories: 347

Day 7	**Total Count:** • Protein: 85 • Carbs: 23g • Fats: 89g • Calories: 1278
Breakfast	**Nice and Juicy Creamed Spinachlings** • Protein: 6g • Carbs: 4g • Fats: 13g • Calories: 157
Snack	**Feisty Chocolate Drizzled Macarrons** • Protein: 2.2g • Carbs: 2.5g • Fats: 6.8g • Calories: 76.5
Lunch	**Skirt Steak With Cilantro Paste** • Protein: 32.3g • Carbs: 2.8g • Fats: 32.5g • Calories: 432

Dinner	**Cheese and Ham Keto Stromboli** • Protein: 25g • Carbs: 9g • Fats: 21g • Calories: 305
Desert	**A Cool Bowl Of Sausage And Cheese** • Protein: 20g • Carbs: 5g • Fats: 16.7 • Calories: 308

Week 3

Day 1	Total Count: • Protein: 149 • Carbs: 64g • Fats: 168g • Calories: 1823
Breakfast	A Carbonara of Pumpkin • Protein: 14g • Carbs: 2g • Fats: 34g • Calories: 2582
Snack	Fantastic Apple Cider Worth Dying For • Calories: 252 • Fat: 0g • Carbohydrates: 30g • Protein: 0g

Lunch	**Pulled Pork Top Of Cornbread Waffles** • Protein: 26.4g • Carbs: 11.7g • Fats: 45.3g • Calories: 556
Dinner	**A Very Low Carb Chicken Satay** • Protein: 105g • Carbs: 18g • Fats: 69g • Calories: 1180
Desert	**Fine Donut Muffins With Sprinkle Sugar** • Protein: 4g • Carbs: 2.5g • Fats: 20.5g • Calories: 210

Day 2	**Total Count:** • Protein: 79 • Carbs: 27g • Fats: 300g • Calories: 249
Breakfast	**Curious Flatbread And Corned Beef** • Calories: 478 • Fat: 25 • Carbohydrates: 3.8g • Protein: 34.2g
Snack	**Tender Soft Pizza Fat Bombs** • Protein: 2.3g • Carbs: 1.5g • Fats: 10g • Calories: 110
Lunch	**Glorious Reversed Bacon Burger** • Protein: 174g • Carbs: 7g • Fats: 207g • Calories: 2597

Dinner	**Slow Cooker Braised Ox Tails** • Calories: 433 • Fat: 30g • Carbohydrates: 5g • Protein: 28g
Desert	**Delightful Choco And Peanut Tart** • Protein: 9.8g • Carbs: 10.5g • Fats: 26.8g • Calories: 304.8

Day 3	Total Count: • Protein: 86.9g • Carbs: 30g • Fats: 178g • Calories: 2172
Breakfast	**Fancy Chicken Roulades Ala Gruyere** • Protein: 42g • Carbs: 2g • Fats: 14g • Calories: 315
Snack	**Beautiful Chocolate Milk Shake With Blackberries** • Protein: 1g • Carbs: 11g • Fats: 34g • Calories: 338
Lunch	**Slow and Crazy Keto Chicken Tikka Masala** • Protein: 26g • Carbs: 6g • Fats: 41g • Calories: 493

Dinner	**Perfectly Braised Short Ribs** • Calories: 550 • Fat: 39g • Carbohydrates: 4g • Protein: 14g
Desert	**A Fine Smoothie Of Blueberry Banana Bread** • Protein: 3.9g • Carbs: 7.6g • Fats: 50g • Calories: 476

Day 4	**Total Count:** • Protein: 149 • Carbs: 64g • Fats: 168g • Calories: 1823
Breakfast	**A Carbonara of Pumpkin** • Protein: 14g • Carbs: 2g • Fats: 34g • Calories: 2582
Snack	**Fantastic Apple Cider Worth Dying For** • Calories: 252 • Fat: 0g • Carbohydrates: 30g • Protein: 0g
Lunch	**Pulled Pork Top Of Cornbread Waffles** • Protein: 26.4g • Carbs: 11.7g • Fats: 45.3g • Calories: 556

Dinner	**A Very Low Carb Chicken Satay** • Protein: 105g • Carbs: 18g • Fats: 69g • Calories: 1180
Desert	**Fine Donut Muffins With Sprinkle Sugar** • Protein: 4g • Carbs: 2.5g • Fats: 20.5g • Calories: 210

Day 5	**Total Count:** • Protein: 79 • Carbs: 27g • Fats: 300g • Calories: 249
Breakfast	**Curious Flatbread And Corned Beef** • Calories: 478 • Fat: 25 • Carbohydrates: 3.8g • Protein: 34.2g
Snack	**Tender Soft Pizza Fat Bombs** • Protein: 2.3g • Carbs: 1.5g • Fats: 10g • Calories: 110
Lunch	**Glorious Reversed Bacon Burger** • Protein: 174g • Carbs: 7g • Fats: 207g • Calories: 2597

Dinner	**Slow Cooker Braised Ox Tails** • Calories: 433 • Fat: 30g • Carbohydrates: 5g • Protein: 28g
Desert	**Delightful Choco And Peanut Tart** • Protein: 9.8g • Carbs: 10.5g • Fats: 26.8g • Calories: 304.8

Day 6	Total Count: • Protein: 86.9g • Carbs: 30g • Fats: 178g • Calories: 2172
Breakfast	**Fancy Chicken Roulades Ala Gruyere** • Protein: 42g • Carbs: 2g • Fats: 14g • Calories: 315
Snack	**Beautiful Chocolate Milk Shake With Blackberries** • Protein: 1g • Carbs: 11g • Fats: 34g • Calories: 338
Lunch	**Slow and Crazy Keto Chicken Tikka Masala** • Protein: 26g • Carbs: 6g • Fats: 41g • Calories: 493

Dinner	**Perfectly Braised Short Ribs** • Calories: 550 • Fat: 39g • Carbohydrates: 4g • Protein: 14g
Desert	**A Fine Smoothie Of Blueberry Banana Bread** • Protein: 3.9g • Carbs: 7.6g • Fats: 50g • Calories: 476

Day 7	**Total Count:** • Protein: 79 • Carbs: 27g • Fats: 300g • Calories: 249
Breakfast	**Curious Flatbread And Corned Beef** • Calories: 478 • Fat: 25 • Carbohydrates: 3.8g • Protein: 34.2g
Snack	**Tender Soft Pizza Fat Bombs** • Protein: 2.3g • Carbs: 1.5g • Fats: 10g • Calories: 110
Lunch	**Glorious Reversed Bacon Burger** • Protein: 174g • Carbs: 7g • Fats: 207g • Calories: 2597

Dinner	**Slow Cooker Braised Ox Tails** • Calories: 433 • Fat: 30g • Carbohydrates: 5g • Protein: 28g
Desert	**Delightful Choco And Peanut Tart** • Protein: 9.8g • Carbs: 10.5g • Fats: 26.8g • Calories: 304.8

Week 4

Day 1	**Total Count:** • Protein: 72 • Carbs: 20g • Fats: 58g • Calories: 1823
Breakfast	**Clean Ham and Apple Flatbread** • Protein: 16g • Carbs: 4g • Fats: 20g • Calories: 1306
Snack	**The Lightning Fast Kimchi Meal** • Protein: 27.3g • Carbs: 9.5g • Fats: 20g • Calories: 334

Lunch	**Pigs In A Blanket** • Protein: 4g • Carbs: 1g • Fats: 6g • Calories: 72
Dinner	**Cute Sausage and Pepper Soup** • Protein: 27g • Carbs: 3.8g • Fats: 2.3g • Calories: 525
Desert	**Soft and Delightful Pumpkin Fudge** • Protein: 1.2g • Carbs: 1.63g • Fats: 10g • Calories: 120

Day 2	Total Count: • Protein: 85 • Carbs: 23g • Fats: 89g • Calories: 1278
Breakfast	Nice and Juicy Creamed Spinachlings • Protein: 6g • Carbs: 4g • Fats: 13g • Calories: 157
Snack	Feisty Chocolate Drizzled Macarrons • Protein: 2.2g • Carbs: 2.5g • Fats: 6.8g • Calories: 76.5
Lunch	Skirt Steak With Cilantro Paste • Protein: 32.3g • Carbs: 2.8g • Fats: 32.5g • Calories: 432

Dinner	**Cheese and Ham Keto Stromboli** • Protein: 25g • Carbs: 9g • Fats: 21g • Calories: 305
Desert	**A Cool Bowl Of Sausage And Cheese** • Protein: 20g • Carbs: 5g • Fats: 16.7 • Calories: 308

Day 3	Total Count: • Protein: 88 • Carbs: 34g • Fats: 152g • Calories: 1925
Breakfast	**A Cool Salad For Early Morning** • Calories: 417 • Fat: 31g • Carbohydrates: 2.55g • Protein: 29g
Snack	**Very Healthy Spinach and Cucumber Mix** • Protein: 3g • Carbs: 7g • Fats: 33g • Calories: 335
Lunch	**Smooth Cauliflower Fried Rice** • Protein: 34g • Carbs: 19.4g • Fats: 48g • Calories: 685

Dinner	**Meatball Of Turky** • Protein: 12g • Carbs: 0.8g • Fats: 10.3g • Calories: 141
Desert	**Cute And Cuddly Vanilla Cloud Muffins** • Protein: 10g • Carbs: 5g • Fats: 30g • Calories: 347

Day 4	**Total Count:** • Protein: 72 • Carbs: 20g • Fats: 58g • Calories: 1823
Breakfast	**Clean Ham and Apple Flatbread** • Protein: 16g • Carbs: 4g • Fats: 20g • Calories: 1306
Snack	**The Lightning Fast Kimchi Meal** • Protein: 27.3g • Carbs: 9.5g • Fats: 20g • Calories: 334
Lunch	**Pigs In A Blanket** • Protein: 4g • Carbs: 1g • Fats: 6g • Calories: 72

Dinner	**Cute Sausage and Pepper Soup** • Protein: 27g • Carbs: 3.8g • Fats: 2.3g • Calories: 525
Desert	**Soft and Delightful Pumpkin Fudge** • Protein: 1.2g • Carbs: 1.63g • Fats: 10g • Calories: 120

Day 5	**Total Count:** • Protein: 89 • Carbs: 33g • Fats: 168g • Calories: 1655
Breakfast	**The Melodious Spring Salad** • Carbs: 6.7g • Fats: 37.3g • Calories: 478 • Protein:: 5g
Snack	**The Most Heart Touching Grand Ma's Hot Chili Soup** • Protein: 28g • Carbs: 10.8g • Fats: 27g • Calories: 395
Lunch	**Delicious Popper Mug Cakes Of Jalapeno** • Protein: 16.5g • Carbs: 8.4g • Fats: 38g • Calories: 429

Dinner	**Authentic Keto Compatible Sushi** • Protein: 18g • Carbs: 5.7g • Fats: 25g • Calories: 353
Desert	**The Mystifying McGriddle Casserole** • Protein: 22.6g • Carbs: 2.9g • Fats: 41g • Calories: 481

Day 6	**Total Count:** • Protein: 50 • Carbs: 17g • Fats: 90g • Calories: 1036
Breakfast	**Great Tomatoes With Poached Up Eggs** • Protein: 16g • Carbs: 5g • Fats: 20g • Calories: 255
Snack	**Pleasing Amaretto Cookies** • Protein: 2.4g • Carbs: 2.5g • Fats: 7.9g • Calories: 85.7
Lunch	**Molten Tuna Bites** • Protein: 6.2g • Carbs: 2.0g • Fats: 11.8g • Calories: 134

Dinner	**Bok Choy Salad With Tofu Tossed In** • Protein: 25g • Carbs: 5.7g • Fats: 35g • Calories: 442
Desert	**Gentle Breeze Strawberry Popsicles** • Protein: 0.5g • Carbs: 2g • Fats: 16g • Calories: 150

# Day 7	**Total Count:** • Protein: 89 • Carbs: 33g • Fats: 168g • Calories: 1655
# Breakfast	**The Melodious Spring Salad** • Carbs: 6.7g • Fats: 37.3g • Calories: 478 • Protein:: 5g
# Snack	**The Most Heart Touching Grand Ma's Hot Chili Soup** • Protein: 28g • Carbs: 10.8g • Fats: 27g • Calories: 395
# Lunch	**Delicious Popper Mug Cakes Of Jalapeno** • Protein: 16.5g • Carbs: 8.4g • Fats: 38g • Calories: 429

Dinner	**Authentic Keto Compatible Sushi** • Protein: 18g • Carbs: 5.7g • Fats: 25g • Calories: 353
Desert	**The Mystifying McGriddle Casserole** • Protein: 22.6g • Carbs: 2.9g • Fats: 41g • Calories: 481

Extra 2 days!

Day 1	**Total Count:** • Protein: 79 • Carbs: 27g • Fats: 300g • Calories: 249
Breakfast	**Curious Flatbread And Corned Beef** • Calories: 478 • Fat: 25 • Carbohydrates: 3.8g • Protein: 34.2g
Snack	**Tender Soft Pizza Fat Bombs** • Protein: 2.3g • Carbs: 1.5g • Fats: 10g • Calories: 110

Lunch	**Glorious Reversed Bacon Burger** • Protein: 174g • Carbs: 7g • Fats: 207g • Calories: 2597
Dinner	**Slow Cooker Braised Ox Tails** • Calories: 433 • Fat: 30g • Carbohydrates: 5g • Protein: 28g
Desert	**Delightful Choco And Peanut Tart** • Protein: 9.8g • Carbs: 10.5g • Fats: 26.8g • Calories: 304.8

Day 2	**Total Count:** • Protein: 86.9g • Carbs: 30g • Fats: 178g • Calories: 2172
Breakfast	**Fancy Chicken Roulades Ala Gruyere** • Protein: 42g • Carbs: 2g • Fats: 14g • Calories: 315
Snack	**Beautiful Chocolate Milk Shake With Blackberries** • Protein: 1g • Carbs: 11g • Fats: 34g • Calories: 338
Lunch	**Slow and Crazy Keto Chicken Tikka Masala** • Protein: 26g • Carbs: 6g • Fats: 41g • Calories: 493

Dinner	**Perfectly Braised Short Ribs** • Calories: 550 • Fat: 39g • Carbohydrates: 4g • Protein: 14g
Desert	**A Fine Smoothie Of Blueberry Banana Bread** • Protein: 3.9g • Carbs: 7.6g • Fats: 50g • Calories: 476

Chapter 1: Breakfast Recipes

Turn Of the Century Caprese Salad

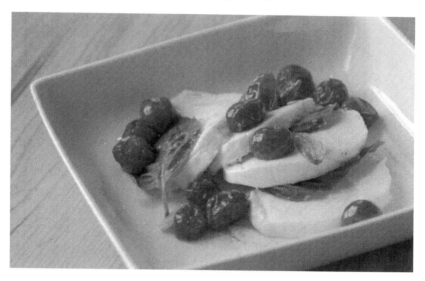

Serving And Preparation Time

The following recipe is going to yield 2 serving and will take about 6 minutes to make and prepare.

Ingredients

- 1 piece of Fresh Tomato
- 6 ounce of Fresh Mozzarella Cheese
- 1/3 a cup of chopped up Fresh Basil
- 3 tablespoon of Olive oil
- Freshly Cracked Black Pepper
- Salt

How To

1. Take a food processor and pulse up your freshly chopped up basil leaves with 2 tablespoon of Olive Oil and turn into a fine paste

2. Slice up your tomatoes into ¼ inch slices

3. Cut up your Mozzarella into 1 ounce slices

4. Assemble your Caprese salad by dishing out layers of tomato, basil leaves and mozzarella

5. Season it up with some extra olive oil, pepper and salt as needed

6. Serve

Nutrition Values

- Protein: 15g
- Carbs: 3.5g
- Fats: 36g
- Calories: 405

The Melodious Spring Salad

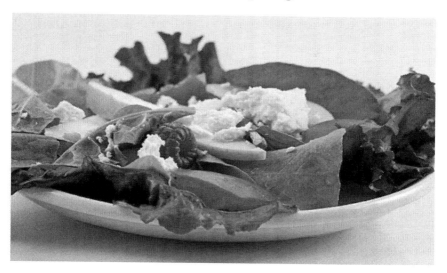

Serving And Preparation Time

The following recipe is going to yield 1 serving and will take about 10-15 minutes to make and prepare.

Ingredients

- 2 ounce of Mixed Green Vegetables

- 3 tablespoon of roasted pine nuts

- 2 tablespoon of 5 minute 5 Keto Raspberry Vinaigrette

- 2 tablespoon of Shaved Parmesan

- 2 slices of Bacon

- Salt as required

- Pepper as required

How To

1. The dish will require you to first take a cooking pan and toss in the bacon.

2. Cook them finely until a nice brown and crispy texture has been achieved

3. Crumble it and toss in the rest of the ingredients into the salad

4. Finely mix it well and if possible, dress it with your favorite dressing and serve

Nutrition Values(Per Serving)

- Protein: 17g

- Carbs: 6.7g

- Fats: 37.3g

- Calories: 478

- Fiber: 2.3g

Great Tomatoes With Poached Up Eggs

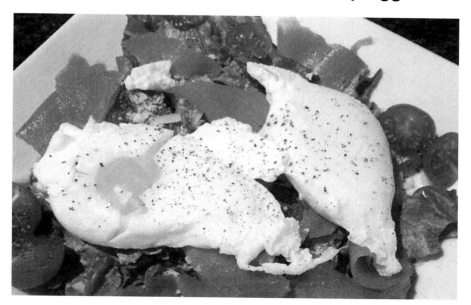

Serving And Preparation Time

The following recipe is going to yield 4 serving and will take about 10 minutes to make and prepare.

Ingredients

Ingredients required for the crust

- 2 cups of grated partially skimmed mozzarella cheese
- ¾ cup of almond flour
- 2 tablespoon of sea salt
- 1/8 teaspoon of dried thyme

Ingredients needed for the topping

- 2 cup of grated Mexican cheese
- ½ of a small onion sliced into thin portions

- ¼ of a medium sized apple. Seeded and cored with the skin intact
- 4 ounce of low carb ham sliced into chunks
- 1/8 teaspoon of dried thyme
- Salt as required
- Pepper as required

How To

1. The first step is to preheat your oven to a temperature of 425 degree Fahrenheit

2. Next, two about two pieces of parchment paper which should be about 2 inches large than a 12 inch pan pizza

3. Prepare a nice double boiler

4. Take a sauce pot and fill it up with just enough water and bring the water to simmer. Once brought to simmer, low down the heat

5. Take the mixing bowl prepared for the double boiler and toss in the cream cheese, mozzarella cheese, almond flour, salt and thyme

6. Gently place the bowl over the simmer pot and keep stirring it continuously while being careful of the steam

7. Once the cheese have melted down and ingredients are combined, pour down the mixture to one of the previously prepared parchment paper and knead it for a few minutes

8. Roll up the whole dough into a ball and place it on the center of the paper

9. Gently keep patting it until a nice circular shape has appeared

10. Cover it with the other parchment paper.

11. Take a rolling pin and keep rolling the dough until it has a nice 12 inch radius

12. Place the prepared dough on a pizza pan and take a fork to drill holes all over

13. Bake it for about 8 minutes

14. Once a golden texture has appeared, lower down the heat to 350 degree Fahrenheit

15. Sprinkle about ¼ cup of the cheese

16. Finely place the sliced onion, apple and ham

17. Bake it again for 5-7 minutes until the cheese has melted and browned

18. Place it on a cooling rack and let it cool for about 3 minutes before cutting into 8 individual slices

Nutrition Values(Per Serving)

- Protein: 16g

- Carbs: 5g

- Fats: 20g

- Calories: 255

Clean Ham and Apple Flatbread

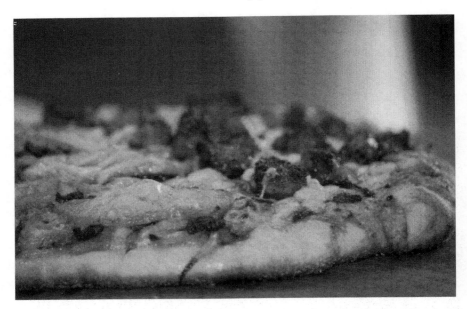

Serving And Preparation Time

The following recipe is going to yield 8 serving and will take about 30 minutes to make and prepare.

Ingredients

Ingredients required for the crust

- 2 cups of grated partially skimmed mozzarella cheese
- ¾ cup of almond flour
- 2 tablespoon of sea salt
- 1/8 teaspoon of dried thyme

Ingredients required for the topping

- 2 cup of grated Mexican cheese
- ½ of a small onion sliced into thin portions

- ¼ of a medium sized apple. Seeded and cored with the skin intact

- 4 ounce of low carb ham sliced into chunks

- 1/8 teaspoon of dried thyme

- Salt as required

- Pepper as required

How To

1. The first step is to preheat your oven to a temperature of 425 degree Fahrenheit

2. Next, two about two pieces of parchment paper which should be about 2 inches large than a 12 inch pan pizza

3. Prepare a nice double boiler

4. Take a sauce pot and fill it up with just enough water and bring the water to simmer. Once brought to simmer, low down the heat

5. Take the mixing bowl prepared for the double boiler and toss in the cream cheese, mozzarella cheese, almond flour, salt and thyme

6. Gently place the bowl over the simmer pot and keep stirring it continuously while being careful of the steam

7. Once the cheese have melted down and ingredients are combined, pour down the mixture to one of the previously prepared parchment paper and knead it for a few minutes

8. Roll up the whole dough into a ball and place it on the center of the paper

9. Gently keep patting it until a nice circular shape has appeared

10. Cover it with the other parchment paper .

11. Take a rolling pin and keep rolling the dough until it has a nice 12 inch radius

12. Place the prepared dough on a pizza pan and take a fork to drill holes all over

13. Bake it for about 8 minutes

14. Once a golden texture has appeared, lower down the heat to 350 degree Fahrenheit

15. Sprinkle about ¼ cup of the cheese

16. Finely place the sliced onion, apple and ham

17. Bake it again for 5-7 minutes until the cheese has melted and browned

18. Place it on a cooling rack and let it cool for about 3 minutes before cutting into 8 individual slices

Nutrition Values(Per Serving)

- Protein: 16g
- Carbs: 4g
- Fats: 20g
- Calories: 255
- Fiber: 1g

Nice and Juicy Creamed Spinachlings

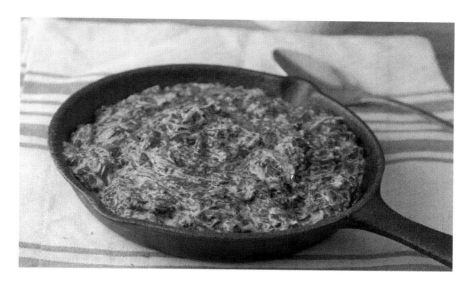

Serving And Preparation Time

The following recipe is going to yield 3 serving and will take about 5 minutes to make and prepare.

Ingredients

- 10 ounce of Frozen Spinach
- 3 tablespoon of Parmesan Cheese
- 3 ounce of Cream Cheese
- 2 tablespoon of Sour Cream
- ¼ teaspoon of Garlic Powder
- ¼ teaspoon of Onion Powder
- Salt as needed
- Pepper as needed

How To

1. Take your frozen spinach and defrost them using a microwave

2. On a pan that is on medium-high heat, toss in the defrosted spinach and let the water boil off

3. Toss in the seasoning alongside the cream cheese to the pan

4. Stir everything together and let the cheese melt

5. Add in the sour cream alongside the parmesan and mix everything well

6. Once the creamed spinach is thickened enough, serve

Nutrition Values

- Protein: 6g
- Carbs: 4g
- Fats: 13g
- Calories: 157

A Cool Salad For Early Morning

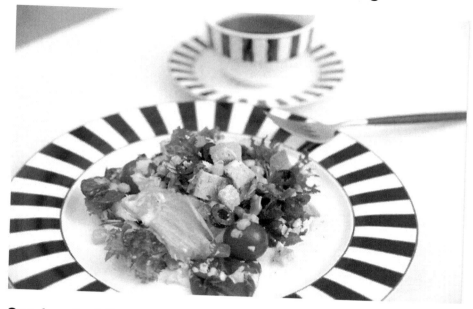

Serving And Preparation Time

The following recipe is going to yield 2 serving and will take about 35 minutes to make and prepare.

Ingredients

- 1 whole piece of chicken

- 1 cup of water

- 1 cup of sour cream

- 1 teaspoon of garlic powder

- 1 teaspoon of black pepper

- 3 cup of baby spinach

- 3 diced up tomatoes

- 1 sliced up avocado

Process

1. The first step is to open up you're the lid of your instant pot and pour in water in your inner pot

2. Toss in your chicken

3. Set the instant pot on poultry mode and let it cook at high pressure for about 30 minutes

4. While that is being cooked, prepare your salad by taking a bowl and toss in the tomatoes, spinach, avocado and finely mix it

5. Toss in your sour cream alongside garlic powder, sprinkled with black pepper

6. By this time, the chicken should be ready. Open up your instant pot and bring it out, only to cut it finely

7. Once cut up, pour in your dressing and serve it warm over your prepared salad.

Nutrition

- Calories: 417
- Fat: 31g
- Carbohydrates: 2.55g
- Protein: 29g

A Carbonara Of Pumpkins

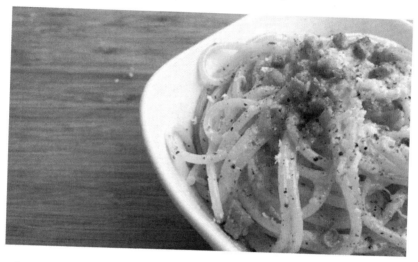

Serving And Preparation Time

The following recipe is going to yield 3 serving and will take about 15 minutes to make and prepare.

Ingredients

- 1 package of Shirataki Noodles
- 5 ounce of Pancetta
- 2 large sized Egg Yolks
- ¼ cup of heavy cream
- 1/3 cup of Parmesan Cheese
- 2 tablespoon of Butter
- 3 tablespoon of Pumpkin Puree
- ½ teaspoon of Dried Sage
- Salt as needed
- Pepper as needed

How To

1. The first step here is to rise off your noodles in hot water for about 2-3 minutes and dry them completely

2. Chop up your pancetta place them in a hot pan.

3. Sear them on the outside and let them get a crispy texture

4. Once done, remove them from the pan and store the fat

5. Take another hot pan and toss in the butter and let it brown

6. Once browned enough, pour in the pumpkin puree and sage

7. Pour in the heavy cream and fat to the mixture and finely mix everything

8. Turn the heat to high and toss in the noodles. Dry fry them for about 5 minutes, you should get a considerable amount of steam.

9. Toss in the parmesan cheese to the pumpkin sauce and mix everything finely

10. Lower down the heat and keep stirring it until a fine thick sauce is produced

11. Toss in the noodles and pancetta into the prepared sauce and toss them well

12. Finally, to top everything off, add in 2 egg yolks and mix them into the sauce

Nutrition Values(Per Serving)

- Protein: 14g
- Carbs: 2g
- Fats: 34g
- Calories: 384
- Fiber: 2g

Curious Flatbread and Corned Beef

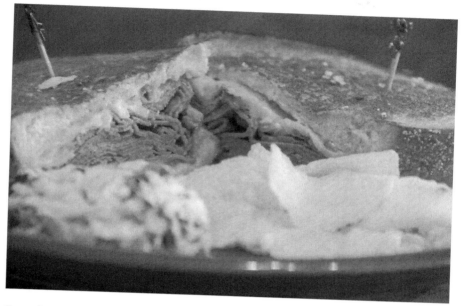

Serving And Preparation Time

The following recipe is going to yield 4 serving and will take about 125 minutes to make and prepare.

Ingredients

- 1 piece of corned beef brisket

- 4 cups of water

- 1 small sized peeled and quartered onion

- 3 cloves of peeled and smashed garlic clove

- 2 pieces of bay leaves

- 3 whole sized black peppercorns

- ½ a teaspoon of allspice berries

- 1 teaspoon of dried thyme

- 5 medium sized carrots
- 1 head of a cabbage cut into wedges

Process

1. First step is to toss in the corned beef, onion, water, garlic cloves, allspice, peppercorn and thymes into your instant pot and close down the lid and set the timer to 90 minutes

2. Once the cooking is complete, turn off your device and allow the pressure to be excreted naturally.

3. Gently take out the meat and place them in a plate, only to cover them up with a tin foil and let it sit for just 15 minutes

4. Toss in the carrots and cabbage to the pot and lock up the lid, letting it cook for 10 minutes

5. Once the cooking is done, release the pressure quickly and take out the prepared vegetables and serve them alongside the corned beef.

Nutrition

- Calories: 478
- Fat: 25
- Carbohydrates: 3.8g
- Protein: 34.2g

Fancy Chicken Roulades Ala Gruyere

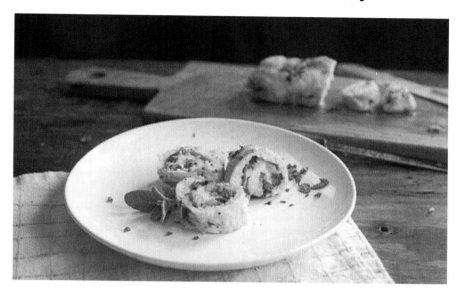

Serving And Preparation Time

The following recipe is going to yield 4 serving and will take about 30-40 minutes to make and prepare.

Ingredients

- 2 pieces of chicken breast
- 1 tablespoon of butter
- 1 medium sized onion all diced up
- 1 tablespoon of white wine vinegar
- 3 ounce of finely grated Gruyere cheese
- 2 tablespoon and a 1 teaspoon of finely chopped fresh sage
- Salt as required
- Pepper as required

How To

1. The first step is to pre-heat your oven to 375 degree Fahrenheit

2. Take a 11 x 13 inch baking pan and line it with parchment paper

3. Take the chicken breast and butterfly them. Take a nice knife and cut it along it side of the breast in a sawing motion. Cut it similar to a opening up a bagel

4. Make sure that you don't completely slice it off, open the breast and lay it flat

5. Sandwich each of the breast between plastic wraps and beat it using a meat tenderizing mallet until they are flat at about ¼ inch thick

6. Season them with pepper and salt

7. Take a medium sized skillet and heat it over medium heat

8. Toss in the butter and let it foam. Toss in the onions and cook them over until they are caramelized

9. Pour in the white wine vinegar and stir in until a syrupy consistency has formed.

10. Remove the heat and toss in the 2 tablespoon of sage and keep stirring it to combine

11. Season with just an amount of pepper and salt

12. Lay out about three pieces of twin and on top of them, place the flattened breast

13. Make sure that the filling is away from the edges, gently spread ½ of the onion mixture over each of the chicken breast

14. Sprinkle about 2 ounce of grated cheese over the breast

15. Gently roll up the breasts and secure them using a twine

16. Take a baking pan and place them in it and sprinkle in the left over sage and cheese over the roulades

17. Bake it for about 35 minutes

18. Remove and let it cool for 5 minutes and serve

Nutrition Values(Per Serving)

- Protein: 42g

- Carbs: 2g

- Fats: 14g

- Calories: 315

- Fiber: 1g

Fan Favorite Pancake

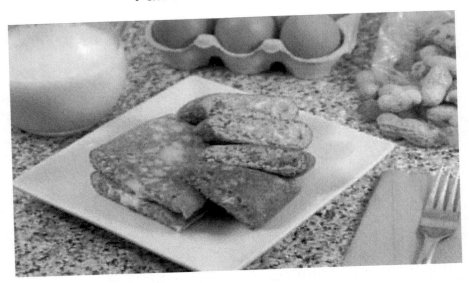

Serving And Preparation Time

The following recipe is going to yield 2 serving and will take about 15 minutes to make and prepare.

Ingredients

For the Peanut Filling
- 1.8 ounce of Fresh Shelled Peanuts
- ½ a teaspoon of Stevia
- Salt as needed

For the Condensed Milk
- ¼ cup of Heavy cream
- 2 drops of Liquid Sucralose

For the Apam Balik
- ½ a cup of Almond Flour
- ½ a teaspoon of Bicarbonate Soda
- ½ a teaspoon of Baking Powder
- 1/8 teaspoon of Salt
- ¼ cup of Almond Milk

- 1 large sized Egg
- 5 drops of Liquid Sucralose
- ½ a teaspoon of Vanilla Extract
- ¼ teaspoon of coconut oil
- 1 tablespoon of Unsalted Butter

How To

1. The first step is to roast up your peanuts and brown them

2. Grind the peanuts alongside the salt and stevia to season it

3. Heat up your heavy cream and sucralose until a nice thick milk has formed

4. Take a mixing bowl and toss in the almond flour, baking powder, salt and baking soda. Mix them.

5. Then in that mixture, pour in the egg sucralose, vanilla extract, almond milk and egg. Mix again

6. Take a pan and melt your coconut oil, and pour in about half of the pancake mix

7. Cover it for about 1 minute and sprinkle in the ground peanuts and spread half of the condensed milk and butter

8. Cover the pan until cooked

9. Repeat until the whole batter is used.

Nutrition(Per Serving)

- Calories: 593

- Fat: 50g

- Carbohydrates: 11g

- Protein: 16g

Old Tale's Bacon Cheddar and Chive Omelet

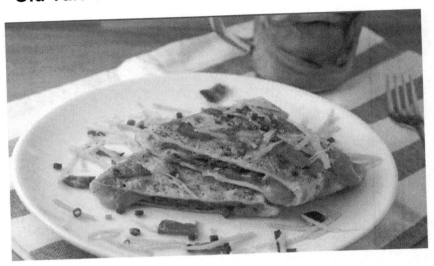

Serving And Preparation Time

The following recipe is going to yield 1 serving and will take about 6 minutes to make and prepare.

Ingredients

- 2 slices of cooked Bacon
- 1 teaspoon of Bacon Fat
- 2 large sized egg
- 1 ounce of Cheddar Cheese
- 2 stalks of Chive
- Salt as needed
- Pepper as needed

How To

7. The first step is to make sure that all of the listed ingredients are prepared. Once done, then take a pan and place it over medium low heat

8. Pour in the bacon fat alongside the eggs and season them with pepper, salt and chive

9. Once the edges start to brown, add in your bacon at the center and let it cook for about 30 seconds before turning off down the stove

10. Pour in the cheese on the top and fold the edges on top of the cheese similar to a burrito,

11. Flip it and gently warm the other side, and you are done!

Nutrition(Per Serving)

- Calories: 463

- Fat: 39

- Carbohydrates: 1g

- Protein: 24g

Beautiful Shrimp and Peanut Curry Dish

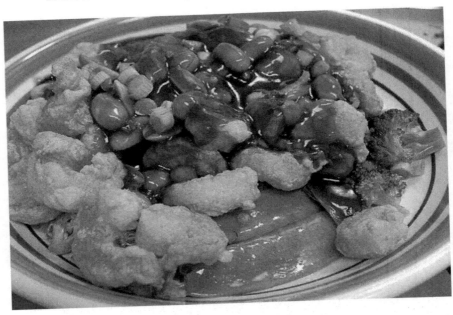

Serving And Preparation Time

The following recipe is going to yield 1 serving and will take about 10-15 minutes to make and prepare.

Ingredients

- 2 tablespoon of Green Curry paste
- 1 cup of vegetable stock
- 1 cup of coconut milk
- 6 ounce of Pre-Cooked shrimp
- 5 ounce of Broccoli florets
- 3 tablespoon of chopped Cilantro
- 2 tablespoon of Coconut Oil

- 1 tablespoon of Peanut Butter
- 1 tablespoon of Soy Sauce
- ½ of a lime juice
- 1 medium sized spring onion chopped up
- 1 teaspoon of crushed roasted garlic
- 1 teaspoon of minced garlic
- 1 teaspoon of fish sauce
- ½ teaspoon of Turmeric
- ¼ teaspoon of Xanthan Gum
- ½ of a cup of source cream

How To

1. Start up by taking a pan over medium heat and add up 2 tablespoon of coconut oil
2. Once the oil is melted toss in the minced ginger and chopped up spring onion. Let them cook for about a minute before pouring the turmeric and curry paste
3. Add about 1 tablespoon of soy sauce, peanut butter and fish sauce and mix them well
4. Then add in a cup of vegetable stock and just a cup of coconut milk.
5. Stir them well before adding the green curry paste.
6. Simmer them for a while
7. Add in about ¼ teaspoon of Xanthan Gum to the curry and mix it properly

8. After a while you will notice that the curry will begin to thicken, that will be the moment when you are going to be needing to throw in the florets and stir them finely

9. Add in the fresh chopped cilantro

10. Once the consistency is fine, you are going to need to toss the weighed pre-cooked shrimp and add the lime juice

11. Let the mixture for a few minutes and season it with pepper and salt as required

12. Finally, serve it hot alongside just a ¼ a cup of sour cream with each serving

Nutrition Values(Per Serving)

- Protein: 27g
- Carbs: 8.9g
- Fats: 31g
- Calories: 454
- Fiber: 4.8g

Chapter 2: Lunch Recipes

Generously Given Nasi Lemak

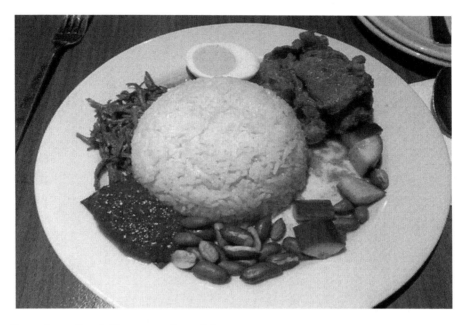

Serving And Preparation Time

The following recipe is going to yield 1 serving and will take about 10 minutes to make and prepare.

Ingredients

- 3 ounce cream cheese
- 3 pieces of large eggs
- 4 tablespoon of Almond Flour
- 1 tablespoon of Coconut Flour
- 1 teaspoon of Baking powder
- 1 teaspoon of Vanilla Extract

- 4 tablespoon of Erythritol

- 10 drops of Liquid Stevia

How To

1. The first step is to toss in all of the ingredients in a bowl and mix them properly using an immersion blender

2. Open up your donut maker and spray it with coconut oil. Pour down the batter on the donut maker

3. Let it cook for about 3 minutes and flip them, let it cook for a more 2 minutes

4. Remove the donuts from the maker and let them cool. Repeat if any batter is left

Nutrition Values(Per Serving)

- Protein: 1.4g

- Carbs: 0.7g

- Fats: 2.7g

- Calories: 32

Delicious Popper Mug Cakes Of Jalapeno

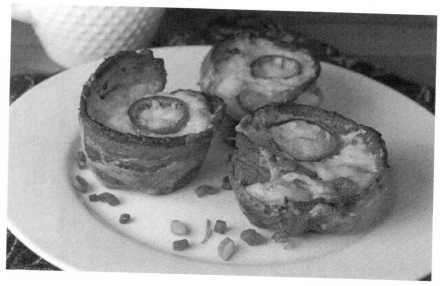

Serving And Preparation Time

The following recipe is going to yield 1 serving and will take about 10 minutes to make and prepare.

Ingredients

- 2 tablespoon of Almont Flour
- 1 tablespoon of Golden Flaxseed Meal
- 1 tablespoon of Butter
- 1 tablespoon of Cream Cheese
- 1 large side Egg
- 1 sliced and cooked bacon
- ½ of a Jalapeno Pepper
- ½ teaspoon of Baking Powder
- ¼ teaspoon of Salt

How To

1. Take a frying pan and place it over medium heat.

2. Take the sliced bacon and cook it until it has a crispy texture

3. Take a container and mix all of the ingredients together

4. Clean the sides

5. Microwave the whole dish for 75 seconds putting it on power 10

6. Gently slam out the cup against a plate to take out the mug cake out

7. Garnish it with some jalapeno and serve it

Nutrition Values(Per Serving)

- Protein: 16.5g
- Carbs: 8.4g
- Fats: 38g
- Calories: 429

Molten Tuna Bites

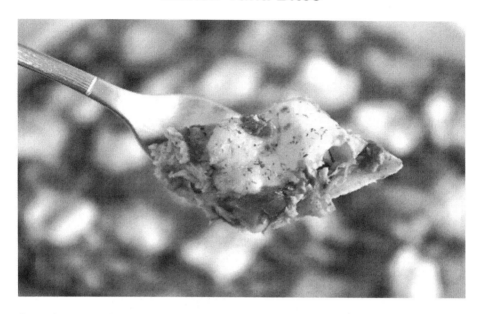

Serving And Preparation Time

The following recipe is going to yield 2 serving and will take about 30 minutes to make and prepare.

Ingredients

- 10 ounce of Drained up Canned Tuna
- ¼ cup of mayonnaise
- 1 cubed and medium sized Avocado
- ¼ cup of Parmesan Cheese
- 1/3 cup of Almond Flour
- ½ teaspoon of Garlic Powder
- ¼ teaspoon of Onion Powder
- Salt as needed

- Pepper as needed
- ½ a cup of Coconut Oil

How To

1. The first step here is to take a mixing bowl and toss in all of the listed ingredients with the exclusion of the coconut oil and avocado

2. Take the cubed avocado and fold them into the tuna

3. Finely tuna into balls and cover them up with Almond Flour

4. Take a pan and pour the coconut oil and heat it up over medium heat

5. Toss in the tuna balls and fry them until a nice brown texture has appeared

6. Serve hot

Nutrition Values(Per Serving)

- Protein: 6.2g
- Carbs: 2.0g
- Fats: 11.8g
- Calories: 134
- Fiber: 1.2g

Pigs in a Blanket

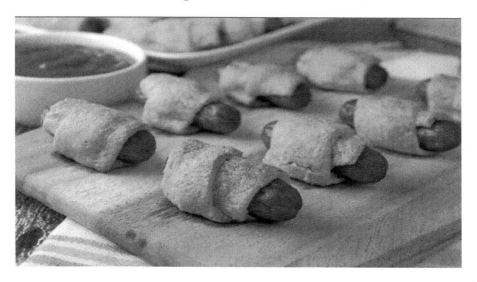

Serving And Preparation Time

The following recipe is going to yield 37 serving and will take about 45 minutes to make and prepare.

Ingredients

- 37 pieces of Little Smokies
- 8 ounce of 2 cups Cheddar Cheese
- ¾ cup of Almond Flour
- 1 tablespoon of Psyllium Husk Powder
- 1 and a half ounce of Cream Cheese
- 1 large sized egg
- ½ a teaspoon of Salt
- ½ a teaspoon of pepper

How To

1. The first step is to measure out all of the wet dry and wet ingredients individually.

2. Take your cheddar cheese and melt it in your microwave In 20 seconds intervals.

3. Once the cheese has started to boil, toss in the ingredients required for the dough

4. Take a silpat and spread out the whole dough all over the sheet and put it inside the fridge for about 20 minutes while you pre-heat your oven to 400 degree Fahrenheit

5. Once cooled, take out the dough to a foil and cut it up. Slice the dough and wrap it around the Smokies

6. Let them for about 15 minutes and then further broil for 2 minutes. Done!

Nutrition Values(Per Serving)

- Protein: 4g

- Carbs: 1g

- Fats: 6g

- Calories: 72

Skirt Steak With Cilantro Paste

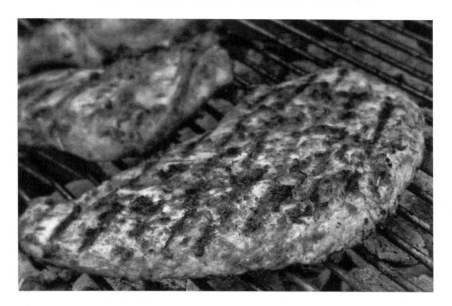

Serving And Preparation Time

The following recipe is going to yield 3 serving and will take about 50 minutes to make and prepare.

Ingredients

For the Cilantro Lime Steak Marinade

- 1 pound of Skirt Steak
- ¼ cup of Soy Sauce
- ¼ cup of Olive Oil
- 1 medium sized lime completely juiced
- 1 teaspoon of Minced Garlic
- 1 small sized Handful Cilantro
- ¼ teaspoon of Red Pepper Flakes

For the Cilantro Paste

- 1 teaspoon of Minced Garlic
- ½ a teaspoon of Salt
- 1 cup of lightly fresh cilantro
- ¼ cup of olive oil
- ½ a medium sized juiced lemon
- 1 medium sized deseeded Jalapeno
- ½ a teaspoon of Cumin
- ½ a teaspoon of Coriander

How To

1. The first step here is to remove outer silver skin off your skirt steak and toss in all of the Cilantro Lime Steak marinade ingredients inside a plastic bag alongside the Steak

2. Let them marinate for about 45 minutes in a fridge

3. For the sauce, you are going to need to toss in all for the paste ingredients to a food processor and pulse them until finely blended

4. Take an iron skillet and put it over medium-high heat

5. Once heated up, toss in the steak to the pan and finely cook on either sides. It should not take more than 2-3 minutes per side

Nutrition Values(Per Serving)

- Protein: 32.3g
- Carbs: 2.8g
- Fats: 32.5g
- Calories: 432
- Fiber: 1g

Smooth Cauliflower Fried Rice

(For Vegetable Lovers)

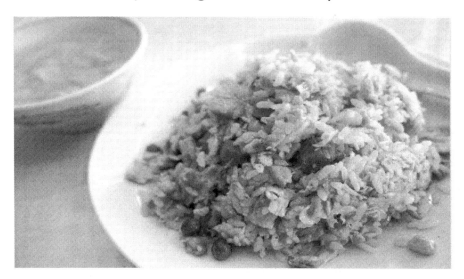

Serving And Preparation Time

The following recipe is going to yield 1 serving and will take about 6 minutes to make and prepare.

Ingredients

- 1 head of grated cauliflower head
- 1 tablespoon of Soy Sauce
- 1 pinch of salt
- 1 pinch of black pepper
- 1 tablespoon of Garlic Powder
- 1 tablespoon of Sesame Oil

How To

1. The first step is to take a food processor and grate your cauliflower

2. Take pan and heat up your oil over the pan

3. Toss in the vegetables, spices, meat and cook them to a desired level of softness

4. Toss in the cauliflower and pour soy sauce for added flavor and color

5. Once done, remove them from the heat and serve.

Nutrition Values(Per Serving)

- Protein: 34g

- Carbs: 19.4g

- Fats: 48g

- Calories: 685

- Fiber: 0.17g

Pulled Pork On Top Of Cornbread Waffles

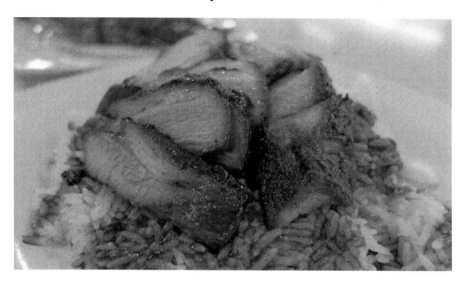

Serving And Preparation Time

The following recipe is going to yield 4 serving and will take about 10 minutes to make and prepare.

Ingredients

- 16 ounce of Pulled Pork
- 1 cup of Almond Flour
- 1 teaspoon of Baking Powder
- ½ a teaspoon of Salt
- 3 large sized egg
- 2 tablespoon of Butter
- ¼ a cup of Sour Cream
- 2 tablespoon of Golden Flaxseed Meal
- 1 tablespoon of Psyllium Husk

- ¼ cup of Coconut Milk

- 2 tablespoon of Chopped up Red Pepper

- ¼ cup of BBQ Sauce

How To

1. The first step is to make the BBQ Sauce (Recipe in this book) and then combine the waffle batter by tossing in all of the wet ingredients into the dry one

2. Open up your waffle iron and pour the batter into the iron

3. While cooking, take a pan and toss in your pork into a pan and pour in about ¾ of your BBQ sauce at medium low heat

4. Once the waffles are complete, spoon up the pork into the waffle and top it with some more BBQ sauce.

Nutrition Values(Per Serving)

- Protein: 26.4g

- Carbs: 11.7g

- Fats: 45.3g

- Calories: 556

- Fiber: 6.1g

Glorious Reversed Bacon Burger

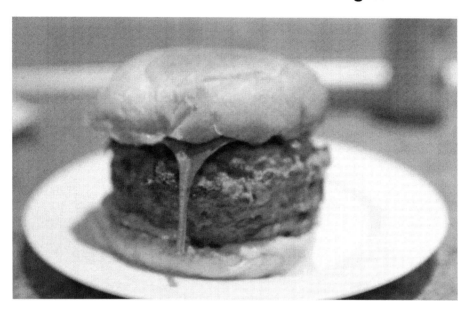

Serving And Preparation Time

The following recipe is going to yield 2 serving and will take about 25 minutes to make and prepare.

Ingredients

- 800g of Ground Beef
- 8 slices of Chopped up Bacon
- ¼ cup of cheddar cheese
- 2 tablespoon of chopped up Chives
- 2 teaspoon of Minced Garlic
- 2 teaspoon of Black Pepper
- 1 tablespoon of Soy Sauce
- 1 and a ¼ teaspoon of Salt
- 1 teaspoon of Onion Powder
- 1 teaspoon of Worcestershire Sauce

How To

1. Take a cast iron skillet and cook up all of your chopped bacon until a fine crispy texture has appeared

2. Once done, remove and place them on a kitchen towel

3. Drain the grease for later use

4. Take a large mixing bowl and toss in the ground beef, 2/3 of chopped up Bacon and the spices

5. Mix the meat finely alongside the spices and form 9 patties

6. Put about 2 tablespoon of Bacon Fat into the cast iron and place the patties once the fat is considerably hot

7. Let them cook for about 4-5 minutes with batches of 3-4

8. Remove them, cool for 5 minutes and top it off with some extra bacon, onion or cheese

Nutrition Values(Per Serving)

- Protein: 174g

- Carbs: 7g

- Fats: 207g

- Calories: 2597

Slow and Crazy Keto Chicken Tikka Masala

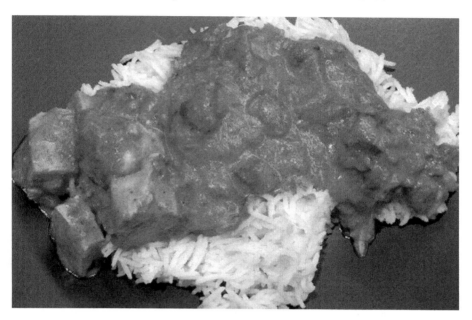

Serving And Preparation Time

The following recipe is going to yield 5 serving and will take about 6 hours to make and prepare.

Ingredients

- 1 and a ½ pound of Chicken Thigh bone in
- 1 pound of Chicken Thigh boneless
- 1 tablespoon of Olive Oil
- 2 tablespoon Onion Powder
- 3 pieces of minced garlic cloves
- 1 inch of grated ginger root
- 3 tablespoon of tomato paste
- 5 teaspoon of Garam Masala

- 2 teaspoon of smoked Paprika
- 4 teaspoon of Kosher Salt
- 10 ounce can of diced up tomatoes
- 1 cu of heavy cream
- 1 cup of coconut milk
- Chopped up Fresh Cilantro
- 1 teaspoon of Guar Gum

How To

1. The first step here is to de-bone the pieces of chicken thighs and chop them up into bite sized portions
2. Toss in the chicken to a slow cooker
3. Take a 1 inch sized ginger knob and grate it over finely
4. Toss in all of the dry spices then
5. Toss in the canned tomatoes alongside the coconut milk and mix them up nicely
6. Let it cook for about 6 hours
7. Once done, mix in the coconut milk, guar gum and heavy cream and finely mix everything
8. Serve hot

Nutrition Values

- Protein: 26g
- Carbs: 6g
- Fats: 41g
- Calories: 493
- Fiber: 2g

Swift Pizza Frittata!

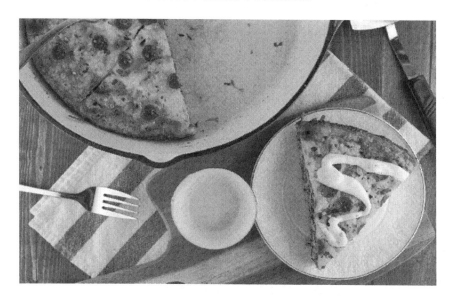

Serving And Preparation Time

The following recipe is going to yield 8 serving and will take about 30 minutes to make and prepare.

Ingredients

- 12 large sized eggs
- 9 ounce of Frozen Spinach
- 1 ounce of pepperoni
- 5 ounce of Mozzarella Cheese
- 1 teaspoon of Minced up Garlic
- ½ a cup of parmesan Cheese
- 4 tablespoon of Olive Oil
- ¼ teaspoon of Nutmeg

- Salt as needed

- Pepper as needed

How To

1. Start off the recipe by microwaving your frozen spinach for about 3-4 minutes

2. Gently squeeze the spinaches later on to drain the water out

3. Pre-heat your oven to a temperature of 375 degree.

4. Take a bowl and mix in the eggs, spices alongside the olive oil

5. Toss in the spinach, parmesan and ricotta

6. Take an iron skillet and pour in the prepared mixture

7. Sprinkle some mozzarella cheese and pepperoni

8. Put it in the oven and let it bake for 30 minutes before serving hot!

Nutrition Values(Per Serving)

- Protein: 20g

- Carbs: 2.1g

- Fats: 23g

- Calories: 298

- Fiber: 20.8

Chapter 3: Dinner Recipes

Sandwich Of Bacon and Healthy Avocado

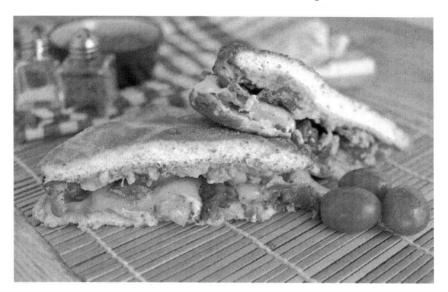

Serving And Preparation Time

The following recipe is going to yield 2 serving and will take about 35 minutes to make and prepare.

Ingredients

Required for the Cloud Bread

- 3 large pieces of eggs
- 3 ounce of cream cheese
- 1/8 teaspoon of tartar cream
- ¼ teaspoon of salt
- ½ teaspoon of garlic powder

Required for the filling

- 1 tablespoon of mayonnaise
- 1 teaspoon of Sriracha

- 2 Bacon slices
- 3 ounce of Chicken
- 2 pepper jack cheese slices
- 2 grape tomatoes
- ¼ of a medium sized avocado

How To

1. First, pre-heat your oven to a temperature of 300 degree Fahrenheit

2. Take three different bowls and crack in the eggs individually

3. Toss in the tartar cream to one bowl alongside some salt and keep whipping until a nice foamy texture appears

4. In another bowl, keep beating the yolk and add in the cream cheese until a fine pale yellow color has appeared

5. Gently pour the egg whites into yolk mixture

6. Take a parchment paper lined baking sheet and scoop about ¼ cup of the prepared batter

7. Finely form them into square shapes and sprinkle just a bit of garlic

8. Bake for 25 minutes

9. On the side, cook the bacon and chicken by seasoning them with some pepper and finally ready the sandwich using the mixture, mayo, halved tomato, mashed avocado, sriracha and cheese.

Nutrition Values(Per Serving)

- Protein: 22g
- Carbs: 4g
- Fats: 28g
- Calories: 361

Authentic Keto Compatible Sushi

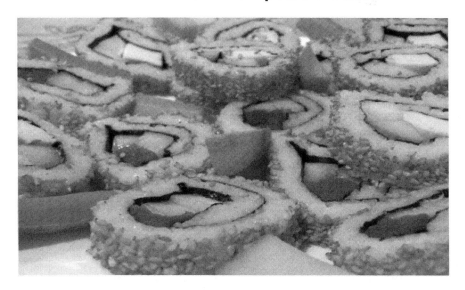

Serving And Preparation Time

The following recipe is going to yield 3 serving and will take about 20 minutes to make and prepare.

Ingredients

- 16 ounce of cauliflower

- 6 ounce of softened cream cheese

- 1-2 tablespoon of Rice Vinegar

- 1 tablespoon of Soy Sauce

- 5 sheets of Nori

- 1 piece of 6 inch cucumber

- ½ a piece of medium Avocado

- 5 ounce of smoked salmon

How To

1. Take a food processor and rice up the cauliflower into rice sized pieces

2. Take a the cucumber and slice it up on each end

3. Gently place the cucumber upright and slice off the sides

4. Finely discard the middle part and slice about 2 pieces into small strips

5. Keep it in a fridge

6. Take a skillet and heat it up, toss in the rice and cook it up

7. Season it with soy sauce

8. Once the cooking is complete, toss the cauliflower to a bowl and mix the cream cheese alongside the rice vinegar

9. Mix well and set it in the fridge

10. Once the mixture is cooled, slice about ½ of your avocado and scoop out small strips out of the shell

11. Take your nori sheet down a bamboo roller and cover it with saran wrap

12. Spread out some cauliflower rice over the nori sheets, toss in the fillings and roll up tightly before serving

Nutrition Values (Per Serving)

- Protein: 18g
- Carbs: 5.7g
- Fats: 25g
- Calories: 353

Bok Choy Salad With Tofu Tossed In

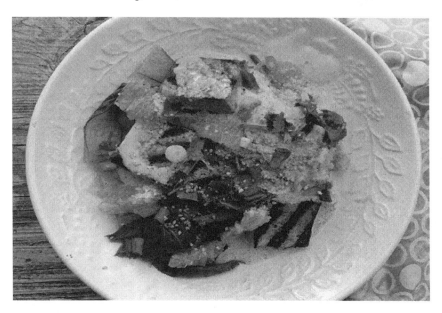

Serving And Preparation Time

The following recipe is going to yield 3 serving and will take about 40 minutes to make and prepare.

Ingredients

For the Oven Baked Tofu

- 150 ounce of Extra Firm Tofu
- 1 tablespoon of Soy Sauce
- 1 tablespoon of Sesame Oil
- 1 tablespoon of Water
- 2 teaspoon of Minced Garlic
- 1 tablespoon of Rice White Vinegar
- ½ a juice of Lemon

For the Bok Choy Salad

- 9 ounce of Bok Choy
- 1 stalk of green onion
- 2 tablespoon of chopped up cilantro
- 3 tablespoon of Coconut oil
- 2 tablespoon of Soy Sauce
- 1 tablespoon of Sambal Olek
- 1 tablespoon of Peanut Butter
- ½ a juice of lime
- 7 drops of Liquid Stevia

How To

1. The first step is to dry press your Tofu for about 5-6 hours
2. Take a bowl and combine all of the ingredients required for the marinade
3. Chop up the tofu into fine square pieces and keep them in a plastic bag alongside the marinade
4. Let it stay overnight for the marinade to settle in
5. Pre-heat your oven to a temperature of 350 degree Fahrenheit
6. Take a nice baking sheet lined with silpat and place the tofu on it
7. Bake for about 30-35 minutes
8. Take another bowl and mix up all of the ingredients needed for salad dressing except the bok Choy, and toss in the spring and cilantro

9. Chop up the processed Bok Choy into small pieces

10. Remove the tofu from your oven and assembled everything together.

Nutrition Values(Per Serving)

- Protein: 25g

- Carbs: 5.7g

- Fats: 35g

- Calories: 442

- Fiber: 1.7g

Cute Sausage And Pepper Soup

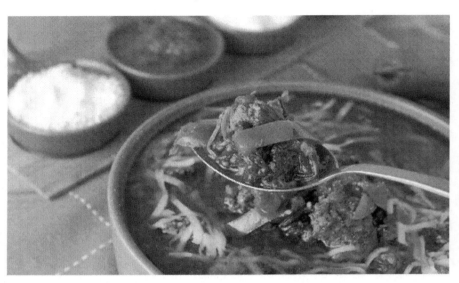

Serving And Preparation Time

The following recipe is going to yield 2 serving and will take about 55 minutes to make and prepare.

Ingredients

- 32 ounce of Pork Sausages
- 1 tablespoon of Olive Oil
- 10 ounce of Raw Spinach
- 1 medium sized Green Bell Pepper
- 1 can of jalapenos with tomatoes
- 4 cup of beef stock
- 1 tablespoon of chili powder
- 1 tablespoon of cumin
- 1 teaspoon of Garlic Powder

- 1 teaspoon of Italian Seasoning
- ¾ teaspoon of Salt

How To

1. The first step is to take a large pot and heat your olive oil over medium heat

2. Toss in the sausages and cook them until seared fine. Stir everything.

3. Slice up the green pepper into fine pieces and toss them to the pot as well

4. Season it with salt and pepper

5. Toss in the tomatoes and jalapenos and mix once more

6. Toss in the spinach on top of everything and close up the lid. Once the spinach is wilted, add in the rest of the spices and broth

7. Close the lid and keep it covered for about 30 minutes over medium low heat.

8. Once done, remove the lid and simmer it for 15 minutes and you are done.

Nutrition Values(Per Serving)

- Protein: 27g
- Carbs: 3.8g
- Fats: 2.3g
- Calories: 525

Cheese and Ham and Keto Stromboli

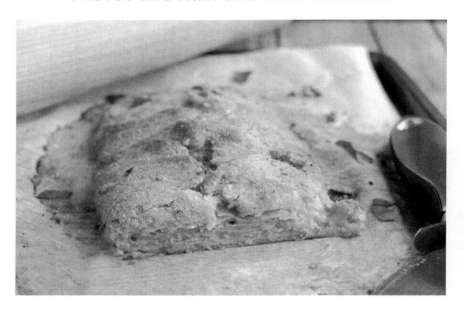

Serving And Preparation Time

The following recipe is going to yield 4 serving and will take about 30 minutes to make and prepare.

Ingredients

- 1 and a quarter cup of shredded mozzarella cheese
- 4 tablespoon of almond flour
- 3 tablespoon of coconut flour
- 1 large sized egg
- 1 teaspoon of Italian seasoning
- 14 ounce of Ham
- 3 and a half ounce of Cheddar Cheese
- Salt as required
- Pepper as required

How To

1. Pre-heat your oven to a temperature of 400 degree Fahrenheit and melt up your mozzarella cheese in a microwave oven

2. Take mixing a bowl and toss in the coconut flour, almond flour and seasoning and mix them properly

3. Then pour in the melted mozzarella cheese and keep mixing

4. After a minute, the cheese will be cooled down and here toss in your egg and mix everything again

5. Once combined, take a fine parchment paper and on a flat surface transfer the mixture

6. Take a rolling pin to flat it out evenly

7. Take a pizza cutter and cut diagonal lines in the dough from the starting from the edges going all the way to the center

8. Make sure that you leave about 4 inches wide rows of the dough untouched in between

9. Between the diagonal layers, fill it up with ham and cheddar

10. Once done, life on section of the dough and roll it on top of another. Completely covering the filling

11. Finally, bake it for about 15-20 minutes and serve when a nice golden brown texture has appeared

Nutrition Values(Per Serving)

- Protein: 25g

- Carbs: 9g

- Fats: 21g

- Calories: 305

Meatballs Of Turky!

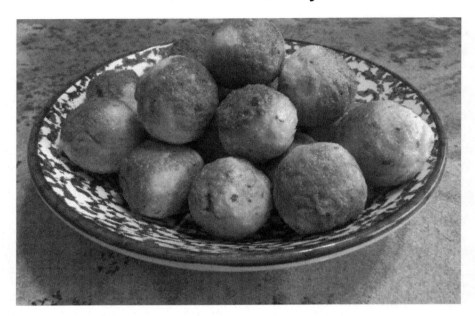

Serving And Preparation Time

The following recipe is going to yield 1 serving and will take about 30 minutes to make and prepare.

Ingredients

- 10 slices of Bacon
- 2 pound of Ground Turkey
- 3 small sized Red Chilies
- ½ a medium green pepper
- 1 small sized Onion
- ½ a teaspoon of Salt
- ½ a teaspoon of Pepper
- 2 large hands of Spinach
- 3 sprigs of Thyme
- 2 large pieces of Eggs
- 1 ounce of Pork Rinds

How To

1. Take a baking sheet cover it with a foil and toss in your bacon

2. Pre-heat you oven to a temperature of 400 degree Fahrenheit

3. Once fully heated, toss in the bacon in your oven and cook for 30 minutes until finely crisped

4. While the bacon is being cooked, take all of the other ingredients and toss them in a food processor and dice them as required

5. Toss in all of the ingredients except the bacon on top of the ground turkey mix and finely mix them

6. Once the bacon is done, take it out and drain the fat

7. Form about 2- meatballs and lay them over the same sheet of bacon

8. Finely Cook up the meatballs for 20 minutes until the juice run clear

9. Skewer about 2-3 pieces of bacon around each meatball

10. Again, take your food processor and combine the bacon fat, spinach, seasoning of your choice and create of stick to serve as a side with your meatball.

Nutrition Values(Per Serving)

- Protein: 12g
- Carbs: 0.8g
- Fats: 10.3g
- Calories: 141
- Fiber: 0.2g

A Very Low Carb Chicken Satay

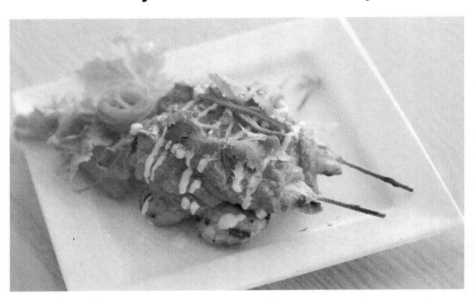

Serving And Preparation Time

The following recipe is going to yield 1 serving and will take about 15 minutes to make and prepare.

Ingredients

- 1 pound of Ground Chicken
- 4 tablespoon of Soy Sauce
- 3 tablespoon of Peanut Butter
- 2 springs of Onion
- 1/3 pieces of Yellow Pepper
- 1 tablespoon of Erythritol
- 1 tablespoon of Rice Vinegar
- 2 teaspoon of Sesame Oil

- 2 teaspoon of Chili Paste

- 1 teaspoon of Minced Garlic

- 1/3 teaspoon of Cayenne Pepper

- ¼ teaspoon of Paprika

- Juice of ½ a lime

How To

1. Heat up about 2 teaspoon of your sesame oil on medium high-heat pan

2. Brown up your chicken and toss in all of the ingredients. Finely mix them and keep cooking

3. Once cooked, toss in about 2 chopped up spring onions and 1/3 of your sliced yellow pepper

4. Serve hot

Nutrition Values(Per Serving)

- Protein: 105g

- Carbs: 18g

- Fats: 69g

- Calories: 1180

Slow Cooker Braised Oxtails

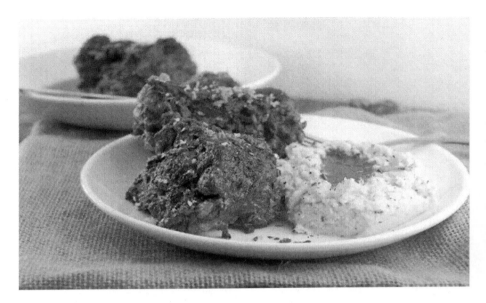

Serving And Preparation Time

The following recipe is going to yield 3 serving and will take about 6-7 hours to make and prepare.

Ingredients

- 2 pound of Oxtails

- 2 cups of beef broth

- 2 tablespoon of soy sauce

- 1 tablespoon of fish sauce

- 3 tablespoon of Tomato Sauce

- 1 teaspoon of Onion powder

- 1 teaspoon of Minced Garlic

- ½ a teaspoon of Ground Ginger

- 1/3 cup of butter
- 1 teaspoon of Dried Thyme
- Salt as needed
- Pepper as needed
- ½ a teaspoon of Guar Gum

How To

1.The first step of this recipe is to pour down your beef broth in a stove and mix it up with your tomato paste, soy sauce, fish sauce and butter and let it heat up

2.Toss in the Ox Tails alongside the seasonings and place it in the cooker

3.Let it cook at low for about 6-7 hours

4.Gently, remove the oxtail from the cooker and set it on a kitchen towel to drain

5.Pour in ½ a teaspoon of Guar Gum to the juice in cooker and use an immersion blender to thicken the juice

6.Serve with a nice side of cauliflower mashed potatoes with the gravy poured in on the top.

Nutrition Values(Per Serving)

- Calories: 433
- Fat: 30g
- Carbohydrates: 5g
- Protein: 28g

Perfectly Braised Short Ribs

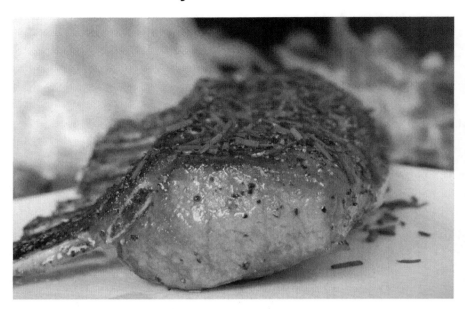

Time to prepare and cook

The recipe will take about 10 minutes to prepare and 35 minutes to cook.

Ingredients

- 4 pound of beef short ribs
- Generous amount of Kosher Salt
- 1 tablespoon of beef fat
- 1 quartered onion with its skin on
- 3 cloves of garlic
- Water

Process

1. Before beginning the cooking, you should first properly season the ribs with your preferred amount of salt

2. Take a skillet and heat up the beef oil over medium high. Toss in the ribs and gently cook them until browned

3. Once browned, toss in the garlic, onion and about 2 inches of water.

4. Once mixed, transfer the mixture to the instant pot and let it cook for about 35 minutes

5. Once the ribs complete, serve the dish with the dish on the bone

6. Alternatively, you can also pull the meat from the bones and braise the liquid and skim the fat. Store them in a jar and serve the ribs with the broth making sure to season them well.

Nutrition

- Calories: 550

- Fat: 39g

- Carbohydrates: 4g

- Protein: 14g

Kung Pao Chicken

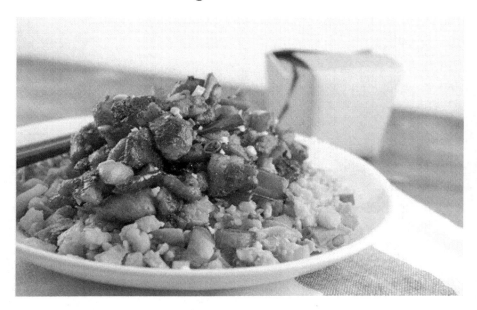

Serving And Preparation Time

The following recipe is going to yield 3 serving and will take about 15 minutes to make and prepare.

Ingredients

For the recipe

- 2 medium sized Chicken Thigh
- 1 teaspoon of Ground Ginger
- Salt as needed
- Pepper as needed
- ¼ cup of Peanuts
- ½ a medium sized Green Pepper
- 2 large sized Spring Onion
- 4 red Bird's eye chilies

For the Sauce

- 1 tablespoon of Soy Sauce
- 2 teaspoon of Rice Wine Vinegar
- 2 tablespoon of Chili Garlic Paste
- 1 tablespoon of Reduced Sugar Ketchup
- 2 teaspoon of Sesame Oil
- ½ a teaspoon of Maple Extract
- 10 drops of liquid Stevia

How To

1. Gently chop up your chicken breast into bite sized portions and season it with ginger, pepper and salt
2. Take you pan and place it over medium-high heat and once the temperature is hot, toss in your chicken and brown them. Should take about 10 minutes
3. Chop up your Chilies and Vegetables and set it aside
4. Ready your sauce by mixing up everything once again
5. When the chicken is properly browned, stir everything together and cook it for another few minutes
6. Toss in the peanuts and vegetables and finally cook them for about 3-4 minutes
7. Finally, add in the sauce and boil it until finely reduced

Nutrition Values (Per Serving)

- Calories: 361
- Fat: 27g
- Carbohydrates: 3.2g
- Protein: 22g

Terrific County Side Gravy

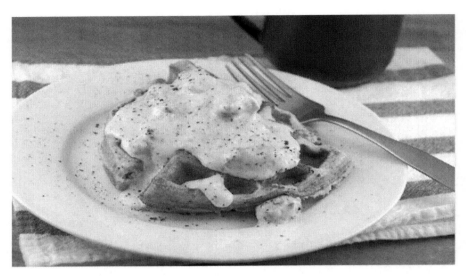

Serving And Preparation Time

The following recipe is going to yield 4 serving and will take about 10 minutes to make and prepare.

Ingredients

- 4 ounce of Breakfast Sausages
- 2 tablespoon of Butter
- 1 cup of heavy cream
- ½ teaspoon of a guar gum
- Salt as needed
- Pepper as needed

How To

1. The first step is to finely toss in the sausages to your heated pan and brown them nicely on all sides

2. Toss in about 2 tablespoon of butter and melt it

3. Pour in the heavy cream and keep stirring it

4. Add in the gar gum and stir it intensely until fully thick

5. Toss in the prepared sausages and stir them gently

6. Serve it to enjoy

Nutrition Values

- Calories: 345

- Fat: 38g

- Carbohydrates: 1.5g

- Protein: 4g

Unlimited Delight Sesame Salmon

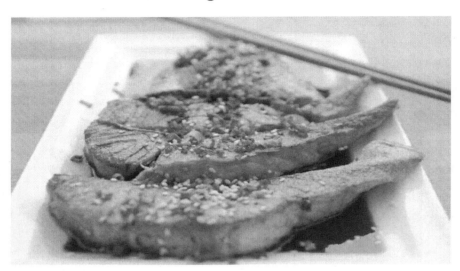

Serving And Preparation Time

The following recipe is going to yield 2 serving and will take about 20 minutes to make and prepare.

Ingredients

- 10 ounce of Salmon Fillet

- 2 tablespoon of Soy Sauce

- 2 teaspoon of Sesame Oil

- 1 tablespoon of Rice Vinegar

- 1 teaspoon of Minced Ginger

- 2 teaspoon of Minced Garlic

- 1 tablespoon of Red boat Fish Sauce

- 1 tablespoon of Sugar Free Ketchup

- 2 tablespoon of White Wine

How To

1.Toss in all of the ingredients to a small sized Tupperware. Just make sure not to toss the sesame oil, white wine and ketchup

2.Marinade everything for about 10-15 minutes

3.Bring down the pan to a nice heat and toss in the sesame oil

4.One the smoke is seen, toss the fish with the skin side down

5.Let it cook until crispy

6.Flip it and cook the other side

7.Each side should take about 3-4 minutes

8.Pour in the marinade liquid to the fish and let it boil

9.Slowly remove the fish from the pan and pour in the ketchup alongside the white wine to the liquid in the pan

10. Simmer for 5 minutes and serve as a side

Nutrition Values(Per Serving)

- Protein: 33g
- Carbs: 2.5g
- Fats: 23.5g
- Calories: 370

Chapter 4: Snacks Recipes

Sinking Boats Of Molten Cheese And Zucchini

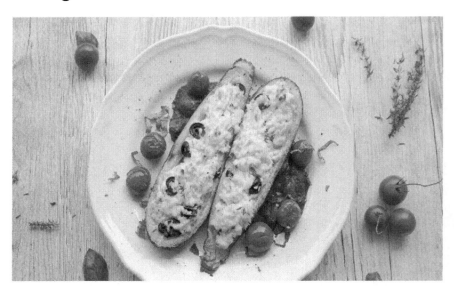

Serving And Preparation Time

The following recipe is going to yield 4 serving and will take about 21 minutes to make and prepare.

Ingredients

- 3 tablespoon of olive oil

- 2 cup of zucchini

- 2 cups of spiralized carrots

- 3 chopped up garlic cloves

- 2 cups of vegetable broth

- 1 tablespoon of black pepper

- 1 tablespoon of garlic powder

Process

1. The first step is to toss in all of the ingredients in your instant pot

2. Cover up the lid and let it cook for about 4 minutes at high pressure

3. Once done, release the pressure naturally and serve it hot with some cheese sprinkled up

Nutrition

- Calories: 237

- Fat: 20g

- Carbohydrates: 7g

- Protein: 10g

The Most Heart Touching Grand Ma's Hot Chili Soup

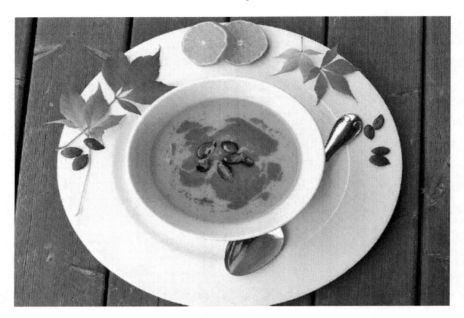

Serving And Preparation Time

The following recipe is going to yield 5 serving and will take about 21 minutes to make and prepare.

Ingredients

- 1 teaspoon of Coriander Seeds
- 2 tablespoon of Olive Oil
- 2 sliced chili pepper
- 2 cups of chicken broth
- 2 cups of water
- 1 teaspoon of Turmeric
- ½ a teaspoon of Ground Cumin
- 4 tablespoon of Tomato Paste
- 16 ounce of chicken thigh

- 2 tablespoon of butter
- 1 medium sized avocado
- 2 ounce of Queso Fresco
- 4 tablespoon of chopped up Cilantro
- Juice of a half lime
- Salt as required
- Pepper as required

How To

1. Cut up your chicken thighs and finely place them in a cooking pan dipped with oil

2. Cook them until brown and place them on the side

3. Tin about just 2 tablespoon of olive oil, toss in the coriander seeds and heat them. Once the fragrance is out, toss in the chili

4. Pour down the water and broth and let it finely simmer

5. Season the mixture with turmeric, pepper, salt and ground cumin

6. Once it has reached a simmering point, add in the tomato paste alongside the butter and stir it to combine and mix

7. Let it simmer for about 10 minutes

8. Pour in the juice

9. In your soup bowl, place about 4 ounces of chicken thighs and ladle it

10. Garnish finally with just ¼ of our avocado and serve it with an ounce of cilantro and queso fresco

Nutrition Values(Per Serving)

- Protein: 28g
- Carbs: 10.8g
- Fats: 27g
- Calories: 395

Pleasing Amaretto Cookies

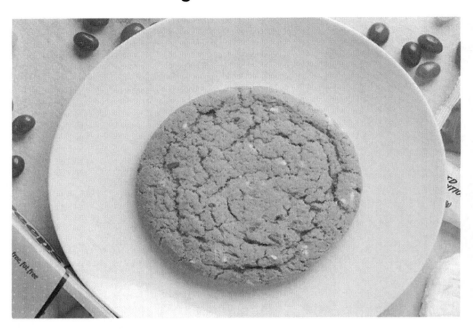

Serving And Preparation Time

The following recipe is going to yield 16 serving and will take about 10 minutes to make and prepare.

Ingredients

- 1 cup of Almond Flour
- 2 tablespoon of Coconut Flour
- ½ a teaspoon of Baking Powder
- ¼ a teaspoon of Cinnamon
- ½ a teaspoon of Salt
- ½ a cup of Erythritol
- 2 large sized eggs

- 4 tablespoon of Coconut Oil
- ½ a teaspoon of Vanilla Extract
- ½ a teaspoon of Almond Extract
- 2 tablespoon of Sugar-Free Jam
- 1 tablespoon of Organic Shredded Coconut

How To

1. Start this recipe off by pre-heating your oven to a temperature of 300F
2. Take 2 muffin tins and spray them with non-sticky spray
3. Take a bowl and toss in the cream cheese, sweetener, egg yolks and vanilla extract.
4. Keep beating them together until they have acquired a nice and smooth consistency
5. Take a separate bowl and gently whip the cream of tartar and egg whites using an electric mixer
6. Gently take the whipped mixture and pour in down into the yolk mixture.
7. Scoop up the mixture and place them in the muffin tins
8. Place the tin inside the oven and let them cook for about 30-35 minutes
9. When done, remove the cakes from the muffin tin and place them on a rack to cool.
10. Take a medium sized and combine all of the ingredients listed under the "Frosting" section

11. Keep beating them using an electric mixer until a smooth consistency has been achieved

12. Fill up the whipped cream in a bag and whip a muffin, place a muffin on top and whip again creating three layers.

13. Serve and eat!

Nutrition Values(Per Serving)

- Protein: 2.4g

- Carbs: 2.5g

- Fats: 7.9g

- Calories: 85.7

- Fiber: 1.3g

The Lightning Fast Kimchi Meal

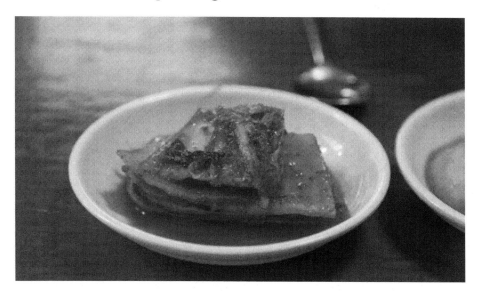

Serving And Preparation Time

The following recipe is going to yield 4 serving and will take about 15 minutes to make and prepare.

Ingredients

For the Quick Kimchi

- 3 cups of Purple Cabbage
- 3 tablespoon of Rice Vinegar
- 1 tablespoon of Minced up Garlic
- 2 teaspoon of minced Ginger
- 1 and a ½ tablespoon of Red Pepper Flakes
- 1/3 of a medium Daikon Radish
- 1 large sized Scallion

- 1 medium sized red Chili
- 1 tablespoon of Red Curry Paste
- 1 and a ½ tablespoon of Soy Sauce

For the Stir Fry

- 1 pound of Pork Tenderloin
- 3 tablespoon of Coconut Oil
- 3 and a ½ ounce of Shitake Mushroom
- 1 large sized Scallion
- 2 tablespoon of White Wine
- 1 tablespoon of NOW Erythritol
- 2 tablespoon of Sesame Oil
- Salt as needed
- Pepper as needed

How To

1. Take your cabbage and slice it up into fine strips

2. Slice up your radish into matchstick sizes

3. Mix up all of the quick Kimchi ingredients in a bowl and combine well

4. Take your pork loin and slice it up to 1/4 inch thick medallions

5. Pour about 1 tablespoon of coconut oil to a pan and toss in half of the pork and cook it until brown spots appear on either sides

6. Repeat for the other half

7.Pour in the wine, 1 tablespoon of coconut oil alongside the sesame oil

8.Toss in the chopped up scallion and shiitake mushrooms and sauté them for about 5 minutes

9.Toss in the Kimchi to the same pan and let the juices boil up for about 4-5 minutes

10. Toss in the pork and cook for a few minutes extra to make sure everything is finely done.

Nutrition Values(Per Serving)

- Protein: 27.3g
- Carbs: 9.5g
- Fats: 20g
- Calories: 334

Feisty Chocolate Drizzled Macaroons

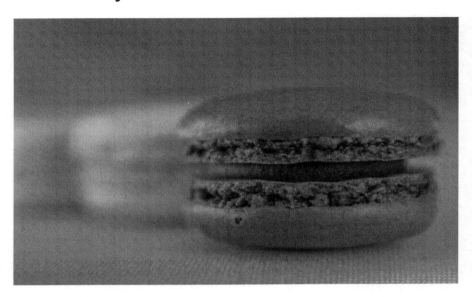

Serving And Preparation Time

The following recipe is going to yield 12 serving and will take about 25 minutes to make and prepare.

Ingredients

- 1 cup of shredded coconut

- 1 large egg white

- ¼ cup of Erythritol

- ½ a teaspoon of Almond Extract

- 1 pinch of salt

- 20g of Sugar free chocolate

- 2 tablespoon of coconut oil

How To

1. The first step here is toe pre-heat your oven to a temperature of 350F

2. Take a parchment paper lined baking sheet and put out a thin layer of coconut

3. Let it bake for about 5 minute until it has been fully toasted.

4. While letting the coconut toast, on the side take a bowl and toss in the eggs. Beat them until foamy texture

5. Add in the salt, Erythritol while mixing the mixture

6. Once the coconut flakes are toasted and cooled down, take them out and toss everything in only to fold them together

7. Take a small ice cream scoop and scoop up the mixture into tight balls of macaroon batter and take them and toss them on the parchment paper

8. Let them bake for about 15 minutes until a golden texture has appeared

9. Once done, drizzle over the molten chocolate and coconut mixture and eat.

Nutrition Values(Per Serving)

- Protein: 2.2g

- Carbs: 2.5g

- Fats: 6.8g

- Calories: 76.5

- Fiber: 1.5g

Very Healthy Spinach and Cucumber Mix

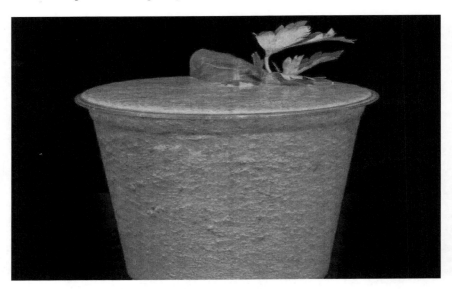

Serving And Preparation Time

The following recipe is going to yield 2 serving and will take about 5 minutes to make and prepare.

Ingredients

- 2 handful of Spinach
- 2.5 ounce of peeled and cubed cucumber
- 7 cubes of Ice
- 1 cup of Coconut Milk
- 12 drops of Liquid Stevia
- ¼ teaspoon of Xanthan Gum
- 1-2 tablespoon of MCT Oil

How To

1. Take a blender and toss in all of the ingredients into the blender

2. Blend it for about 1-2 minutes until everything is finely mixed

3. Serve

Nutrition Values(Per Serving)

- Protein: 3g

- Carbs: 7g

- Fats: 33g

- Calories: 335

- Fiber: 3g

Fantastic Apple Cider Worth Dying For

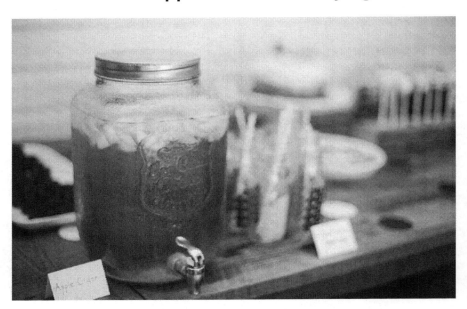

Time to prepare and cook

The recipe will take about 5 minutes to prepare and 6 minutes to cook with 4 servings

Ingredients

- 2 cups of moderately dry white wine
- ½ a cup of sugar
- ¼ teaspoon of grated nutmeg
- 1 piece of 4 inch cinnamon stick
- 8 whole cloves
- 4 pieces of large firm apples

Process

1. Take your wine, sugar, cinnamon stick, nutmeg and cloves in your instant pot and sauté them until the sugar dissolves

2. Toss in your halved apples then and lock up the lid

3. Let it cook at high pressure for 6 minutes

4. Quick release the pressure

5. Unlock the pot and transfer the halves to a bowl

6. Bring the sauce in the pot to a medium heat and cook for 5 minutes, stirring it until the syrup is thickened

7. Discard the cinnamon sticks and cloves and pour the syrup over your apples

Nutrition

- Calories: 252

- Fat: 0g

- Carbohydrates: 30g

- Protein: 0g

Tender Soft Pizza Fat Bombs

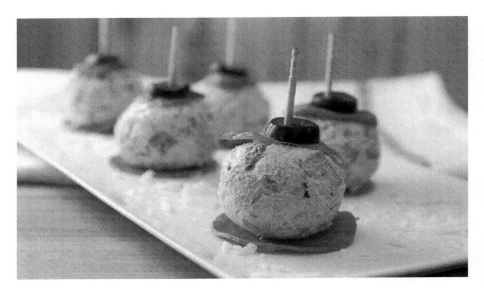

Serving And Preparation Time

The following recipe is going to yield 6 serving and will take about 15 minutes to make and prepare.

Ingredients

- 4 ounce of cream cheese
- 14 slices of peperoni
- 8 pitted of black Olives
- 2 tablespoon of Sun Dried Tomato Pesto
- 2 tablespoon of chopped of Fresh Basil
- Salt as needed
- Pepper as needed

How To

1. The first step of this fairly easy recipe is to dice up your olives and pepperonis to fine small sizes

2. Toss in all of the other ingredients and mix it up

3. Form fine balls and garnish them up with olive, pepperoni and basil

Nutrition Values

- Protein: 2.3g

- Carbs: 1.5g

- Fats: 10g

- Calories: 110

- Fiber: 0.2g

Beautiful Chocolate Milk Shake With Blackberries

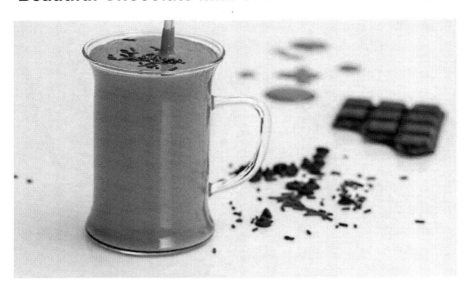

Serving And Preparation Time

The following recipe is going to yield 2 serving and will take about 5 minutes to make and prepare.

Ingredients

- 7 cubes of ice

- 1 cup of unsweetened coconut milk

- ¼ cup of blackberries

- 2 tablespoon of Cocoa Powder

- 12 drops of Liquid Stevia

- ¼ teaspoon of Xanthan Gum

- 1-2 tablespoon of MCT Oil

How To

1. Take a blender and toss in all of the ingredients into the blender

2. Blend it for about 1-2 minutes until everything is finely mixed

3. Serve

Nutrition Values(Per Serving)

- Protein: 1g

- Carbs: 11g

- Fats: 34g

- Calories: 338

- Fiber: 7g

Happily Ever After Tater Tots

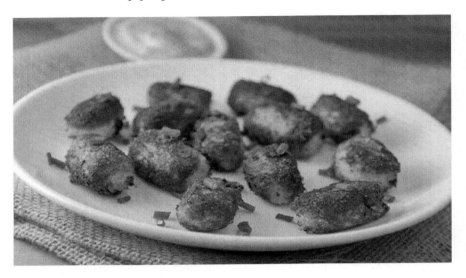

Serving And Preparation Time

The following recipe is going to yield 4 serving and will take about 10 minutes to make and prepare.

Ingredients

- 1 medium sized Cauliflower Head
- ¼ cup of grated Parmesan Cheese
- 2 ounce of Shredded Mozzarella Cheese
- 1 large sized egg
- ½ a teaspoon of Onion Powder
- ½ a teaspoon of Garlic Powder
- 2 teaspoon of Psyllium Husk Powder
- Salt as needed
- Pepper as needed
- 1 cup of Bacon Fat

How To

1. Cup of the heads of the cauliflower into nice florets and steam it until soft

2. Pulse them in a food processor until completely mashed

3. Cool the cauliflower and put them in a dish cloth to squeeze out excess water

4. Toss in the egg, cheese and other spices

5. Mix everything together until finely thick

6. Toss in the phylum husk

7. Roll batter into fine tater tots

8. Take a pan and heat up the oil

9. Fry them until browned

10. Lay them on a kitchen towel and serve

Nutrition Values

- Protein: 10g

- Carbs: 9g

- Fats: 21g

- Calories: 248

Lovely Potato Gratin

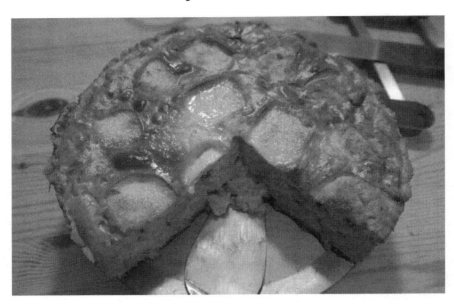

Time to prepare and cook

The recipe will take about 10 minutes to prepare and 9 minutes to cook

Ingredients

- 3 tablespoon of olive oil

- 3 cups of sliced up parsnips

- 3 cloves of chopped up garlic

- 2 cups of vegetable broth

- 1 tablespoon of black pepper

- 1 tablespoon of garlic powder

- 1 cup of cream cheese

- 2 cups of mozzarella cheese

Process

1. The first step here is to toss in all of your ingredients in the instant pot's inner pot except the cheddar cheese

2. Close up the lid and let it cook at high pressure for 5 minutes

3. Wait for about 10 minutes and let the pressure release naturally

4. Open up the lid and sprinkle mozzarella cheese all over

5. Set the instant pot to warm settings for about 5 minutes for the cheese to melt

6. Serve hot

Nutrition

- Calories: 201

- Fat: 10g

- Carbohydrates: 22g

- Protein: 6g

Fried Kale Sprouts

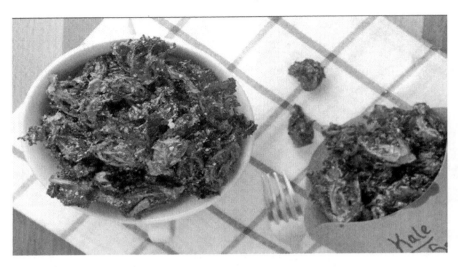

Serving And Preparation Time

The following recipe is going to yield 2 serving and will take about 10 minutes to make and prepare.

Ingredients

- ½ a bag of Kale Sprouts
- Oil as needed
- 2 tablespoon of Parmesan Cheese
- Salt as required
- Pepper as required

How To

7. Take a pan and pour in some oil and heat it up
8. Toss in the kale sprouts in the fryer
9. Fry the sprouts until nicely browned on the edge of the bulb

10. Once done, remove them place them on a kitchen towel to drain off the excess grease

11. Season them finely and serve

Nutrition Values(Per Serving)

- Calories: 108
- Fat: 9g
- Carbohydrates: 5g
- Protein: 4g

Chapter 5: Desert Recipes

Cheddar and Cheese Waffles To Die For

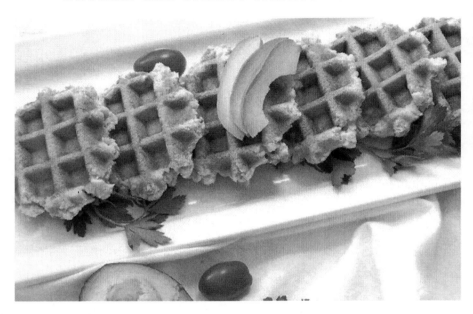

Serving And Preparation Time

The following recipe is going to yield 12 serving and will take about 20 minutes to make and prepare.

Ingredients

- 1 and a 1/3 cup of sifted coconut flour
- 3 teaspoon of baking powder
- 1 teaspoon of dried ground sage
- ½ a teaspoon of salt
- ¼ a teaspoon of garlic powder
- 2 cups of canned coconut milk
- ½ a cup of water

- 2 pieces of egg
- 3 tablespoon of melted coconut oil
- 1 cup of shredded cheddar cheese

How To

1. The first step is to heat up your waffle iron and set it to a moderate heat settings

2. Take a mixing bowl and toss in the baking powder, seasoning and flour and whisk them altogether nicely

3. Pour down all of the liquid ingredients and keep stirring until a nice batter forms

4. Toss in the cheese

5. Next up, open up your waffle iron and grease up the top and bottom sides

6. In about the waffle container, gently scoop of about 1/3 of the batter and pour it in the iron sections

7. Close down the Iron and let it cook until steam starts to rise from the top

8. Once done, open up your waffle iron and take out the waffles, to serve them hot.

9. Usually you are going to need about 2 cycles of moderate heat to cook them properly

Nutrition Values(Per Serving)

- Protein: 6g
- Carbs: 3.81g
- Fats: 17g
- Calories: 213

The Mystifying McGriddle Casserole

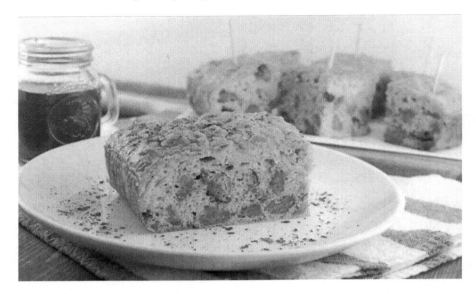

Serving: 8

Prep Time: 15 minutes

Cook Time: 40 minutes

Ingredients

- 1 cup of almond flour
- ¼ cup of Flaxseed Meal
- 1 pound of breakfast sausage
- 10 large pieces of eggs
- 4 ounce of cheddar cheese
- 6 tablespoon of Walden Farms Maple Syrup
- 4 tablespoon of Butter
- ½ a teaspoon of Onion Powder

- ½ a teaspoon of Garlic Powder
- ¼ teaspoon of Sage
- Salt as required
- Pepper as required

How To

1. Pre-heat your oven to a temperature of 350 degree Fahrenheit
2. Take your pan and put in your stove over medium heat and toss in the breakfast sausage and break it up while cooking
3. Take a separate bowl and in that bowl, toss in all the dry ingredients and then toss in all of the wet ingredients
4. Toss in just 4 tablespoon of syrup and mix everything finely
5. Once the sausage are browned, pour in the mixture and mix again a little bit more
6. Prepare a 9x9 casserole dish using a parchment paper and pour in the casserole mixture in the dish
7. Use 2 table spoon and drizzle them over the final mixture
8. Place it in the oven and let it bake for about 45-55 minutes
9. Remove it slowly lift It out, and serve

Nutrition Values(Per Serving)

- Protein: 22.6g
- Carbs: 2.9g
- Fats: 41g
- Calories: 481
- Fiber: 2.5g

Gentle Breeze Strawberry Popsicles

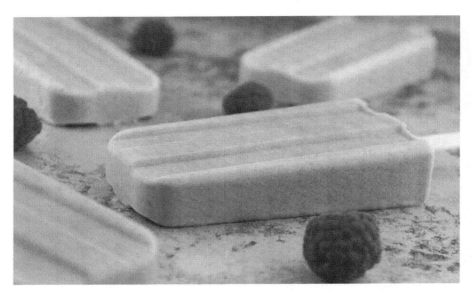

Serving: 6

Prep Time: 10 minutes

Cook Time: 120 minutes

Ingredients

- 100g of Raspberries
- Juice of ½ a lemon
- ¼ cup of coconut oil
- 1 cup of coconut milk
- ¼ cup of sour cream
- ¼ cup of heavy cream
- ½ a teaspoon of Guar Gum
- 20 drops of Liquid Stevia

How To

1.Take an immersion blender and toss in all of the ingredients and blend them altogether nicely

2.Once done, take them mixture through a mesh and strain the mixture, discarding all of the raspberry seeds

3.Pour in the mixture into a mold and keep the mold inside the fridge for 2 hours

4.Once done, pass the mold through hot water to dislodge the popsicles

Nutrition Values(Per Serving)

- Protein: 0.5g
- Carbs: 2g
- Fats: 16g
- Calories: 150

Soft and Delightful Pumpkin Fudge

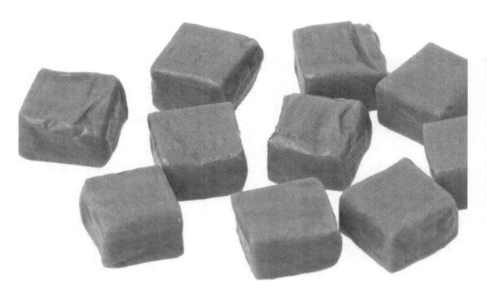

Serving And Preparation Time

The following recipe is going to yield 25 serving and will take about 1-2 hours to make and prepare.

Ingredients

- 1 and a ¾ cup of coconut butter
- 1 cup of pumpkin puree
- 1 teaspoon of ground cinnamon
- ¼ teaspoon of ground nutmeg
- 1 tablespoon of coconut oil

How To

1. Take a 8x8 inch square baking pan and line it with aluminum foil to start with

2. Take a spoon of scoop up the coconut butter into a heated pan and let the butter melt over low heat

3. Keep stirring it and remove the heat gently

4. Toss in the spices and pumpkin and keep stirring it until a grainy texture has formed

5. Pour in the coconut oil and keep stirring it vigorously in order to make sure that everything is combined nicely

6. Scoop up the mixture into the previously prepared baking pan and distribute evenly

7. Place a piece of wax paper over the top of the mixture and press on the upper side to make evenly straighten up the topside

8. Remove the wax paper and throw it away

9. Place the mixture into your fridge and let it cool for about 1-2 hours

10. Take it out and cut it into slices, then eat

Nutrition Values

- Protein: 1.2g
- Carbs: 1.63g
- Fats: 10g
- Calories: 120
- Fiber: 2.61g

A Cool Bowl of Sausage And Cheese

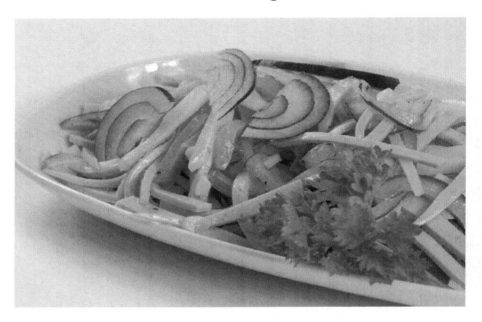

Serving And Preparation Time

The following recipe is going to yield 1 serving and will take about 40 minutes to make and prepare.

Ingredients

- 1 and a ½ of cheddar and bacon chicken sausage
- ¾ of cup grated cheddar cheese
- ¼ cup of coconut flour
- ¼ cup of coconut oil
- 2 tablespoon of coconut milk
- 5 pieces of egg yolks
- 2 teaspoon of Lemon Juice
- ½ a teaspoon of Rosemary
- ¼ teaspoon of Cayenne Pepper
- ¼ teaspoon of Baking Soda
- 1/8 teaspoon of Salt

How To

1. The first thing you have to do is cube up your chicken sausage into small sizes

2. Fry them up over medium heat

3. Pre-heat your temperature to 350 degree Fahrenheit

4. Separate the 5 egg yolks from your eggs and discard the whites

5. Finely measure out the dry flours and spices alongside the bowl

6. Mix up all of the dry ingredients and combine them

7. Beat the egg yolk until foamy for about 4-5 minutes

8. Pour in the coconut oil, lemon juice, coconut milk and keep beating it

9. Pour in the wet ingredients and mix it with the dry ingredients nicely

10. Fold about ½ a cup of cheddar cheese into the batter

11. Take 2 ramekins and fill them up using the mixture about 3/4th of the way

12. In the meantime, the sausages should be ready. Poke them into your batter and finally bake the mixture for 20-25 minutes until nicely browned

13. Server and eat

Nutrition Values(Per Serving)

*   Protein: 20g
*   Carbs: 5g
*   Fats: 16.7
*   Calories: 308
*   Fiber: 2g

Cute and Cuddly Vanilla Cloud Muffins

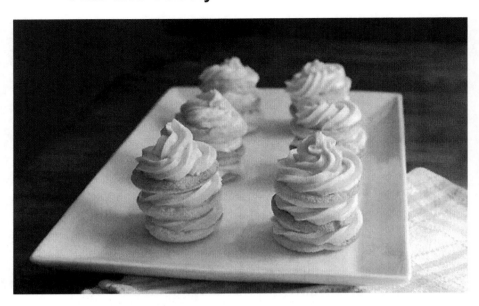

Serving And Preparation Time

The following recipe is going to yield 8 serving and will take about 55 minutes to make and prepare.

Ingredients

For the cake
- 6 pieces of large separated large eggs
- 6 tablespoon of cream cheese at room temperature
- ½ a teaspoon of tartar cream
- 2 teaspoon of vanilla extract
- ¼ cup of granulated stevia

For the Frosting
- 16 ounce of softened cream cheese
- 2 tablespoon of butter
- 1/3 cup of granulated stevia
- 1 tablespoon of vanilla extract

How To

1. Pre-heat your oven to a temperature of 300 degree Fahrenheit

2. Take about 2 muffin tins and grease them with spray oil

3. Take a medium sized bowl and toss in the cream cheese, sweetener, egg yolks, vanilla extract until a nice smooth consistency has been achieved

4. Take another bowl, and whip the tartar cream and egg whites using an mixer until a foam appears

5. Then, gently pour in the whites mixture to the yolk mixture

6. Scoop up about 2 tablespoon of the mixture into each of the muffin tins

7. Place it in the oven for 30-35 minutes until browned

8. Take them out and let it cool on a cooling rack

9. Take another bowl and mix in all the ingredients of the frosting and beat with a mixer

10. Move the frosting into a pastry bag and put a layer of frosting between on top a cake, and put another cake on top of the frosting. Make a total of three layers.

Nutrition Values(Per Serving)

- Protein: 10g

- Carbs: 5g

- Fats: 30g

- Calories: 347

Fine Donut Muffins With Sprinkled Sugar

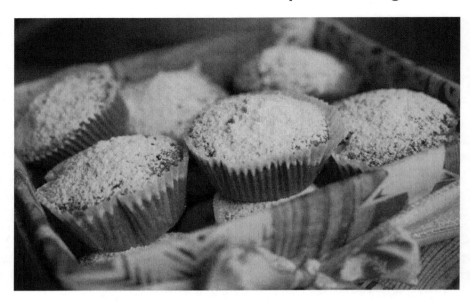

Serving And Preparation Time

The following recipe is going to yield 12 serving and will take about 35-40 minutes to make and prepare.

Ingredients

For the Donut Muffin

- 1 and a ½ cup of Almond Flour

- ½ a cup of powdered Erythrtiol

- 2 tablespoon of Psyllium Husk Powder

- ½ a cup of Heavy Cream

- 1/3 cup of Heavy Cream

- 2 large sized eggs

- 1 and a ½ teaspoon of Baking Powder

- 12 a teaspoon of Orange Extract
- ¼ teaspoon of Nutmeg
- ¼ teaspoon of Allspice
- ¼ teaspoon of Liquid Stevia
- 1/8 teaspoon of Ground Clove
- 1/8 teaspoon of Ground Ginger

For the Sugar Coating

- ¼ cup of molten Butter
- ¼ cup of Erythritol
- 1 teaspoon of Cinnamon
-

How To

1. Toss in your butter in a saucepan and brown it over medium-low heat
2. Powder your Erythritol and clove twig by tossing them in a spice grinder
3. Mix up all of the dry ingredients then.
4. Once your butter is browned, cool it down and toss in all of the wet ingredients to a bowl and mix it using a mixer
5. Sift about ½ of the dry ingredients into the wet ingredients mixture and repeat it once again until a fine dough is generated
6. Pre-heat your oven to a temperature of 350 degree Fahrenheit

7. Divide the dough into 12 silicon cupcake containers and bake for 20-25 minutes

8. Melt up about ¼ cup of your butter and toss them in your saucepan

9. Combine the cinnamon and sweeteners

10. Dip the muffins in to the butter and then into the sweet mixture and garnish with your favorite toppings before serving.

Nutrition Values(Per Serving)

- Protein: 4g
- Carbs: 2.5g
- Fats: 20.5g
- Calories: 210
- Fiber: 2.7g

Delightful Choco And Peanut Tart

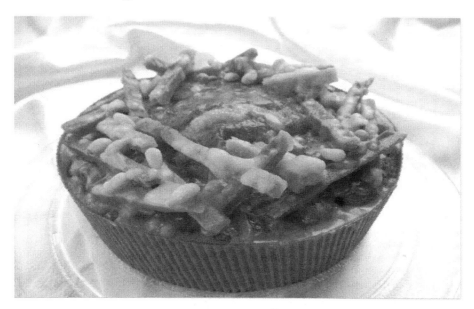

Serving And Preparation Time

The following recipe is going to yield 4 serving and will take about 15 minutes to make and prepare.

Ingredients

For The Crust

- ¼ cup of Flaxseed

- 2 tablespoon of Almond Flour

- 1 tablespoon of Erythritol

- 1 Large Egg White

For The Top Layer

- 1 Medium sized Avocado

- 4 tablespoon of Cocoa Powder

- ¼ cup of Erythritol
- ½ teaspoon of vanilla extract
- ½ teaspoon of Cinnamon
- 2 tablespoon of Heavy Cream

Middle Layer

- 4 tablespoon of Peanut Butter
- 2 tablespoon of butter

How To

1. Preheat our oven to a temperature of 350F

2. Take a separate bowl and toss in the flaxseed and grind them until they are firmly grounded

3. To the flaxseed mix, add up the rest of the ingredients listed under crust

4. Take a tart pan and pour down the crust mixture and put it inside the oven and bake it for 8 minutes

5. Take another bowl and prepare the top layer by combining all of the ingredients listed under crust and blend them to get a creamy and smooth mixture.

6. Once the curst inside the oven is complete, take it out and let it cool

7. For the peanut butter layer, you are going to need to take another bowl and melt the peanut butter and butter mixture in your microwave.

8. Gently pour down the molten Peanut butter mixture on top of your crust letter and leave it for 30 minutes to settle down

9. Over the Peanut Butter layer, pour down the chocolate avocado layer and let the whole tart refrigerate for an hour.

10. Take It out from the fridge and serve them well.

Nutrition Values(Per Serving)

- Protein: 9.8g

- Carbs: 10.5g

- Fats: 26.8g

- Calories: 304.8

- Fiber: 6.6g

A Fine Smoothie Of Blueberry Banana Bread

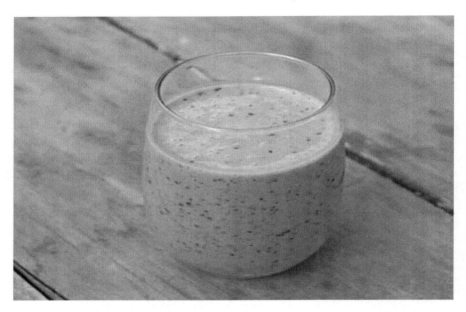

Serving And Preparation Time

The following recipe is going to yield 2 serving and will take about 5 minutes to make and prepare.

Ingredients

- 3 tablespoon of Golden Flaxseed Meal

- 1 tablespoon of Chia Seeds

- 2 cups of Unsweetened Coconut Milk

- 10 drops of Liquid Stevia

- ¼ cup of Blueberries

- 2 tablespoon of MCT Oil

- 1 and a ½ teaspoon of Banana Extract

- ¼ a teaspoon of Xanthan Gum

How To

1. Take a blender and toss in all of the ingredients into the blender

2. Take a few moments and let the flax and chia seeds settle in

3. Blend it for about 1-2 minutes until everything is finely mixed

4. Serve

Nutrition Values(Per Serving)

- Protein: 3.9g

- Carbs: 7.6g

- Fats: 50g

- Calories: 476

- Fiber: 1g

Adorable Tartlets

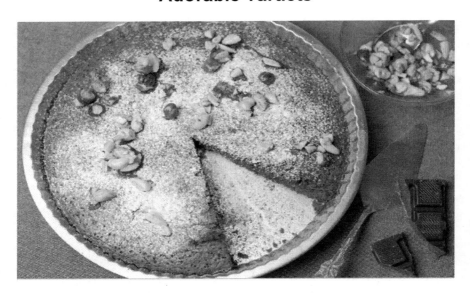

Serving And Preparation Time

The following recipe is going to yield 1 serving and will take about 30 minutes to make and prepare.

Ingredients

For the Pastry

- 1 cup of Almond Flour
- 3 tablespoon of Coconut Flour
- 5 tablespoon of Butter
- ¼ teaspoon of Salt
- 1 teaspoon of Xanthan Gum
- 1 teaspoon of Oregano
- ¼ teaspoon of Paprika

- ¼ teaspoon of Cayenne
- 2 tablespoon of Ice Water

For the Filling

- 1/3 cup of Cheese
- 400g of Ground Beef
- 80g of Mushroom
- 3 stalks of Spring Onion
- 2 tablespoon of Tomato Paste
- 2 tablespoon of Tomato Paste
- 1 tablespoon of Olive Oil
- 2 teaspoon of Yellow Mustard
- 2 teaspoon of Garlic
- 1 teaspoon of Cumin
- ½ a teaspoon of Pepper
- 1 teaspoon of Salt
- 1 teaspoon of Worcestershire Sauce
- ¼ teaspoon of Cinnamon

How To

1. Start off your recipe by mixing up all of the dry ingredients for the pastry and tossing them in a food processor

2. Chop off cold butter into your food processor as well and pulse everything until finely crumbly. If consistency seems off, then add 1 tablespoon of water

3. Chill out your dough in a fridge for about 10 minutes

4. Take the dough and using 2 silpats, roll the dough in between using a rolling pin

5. Take a cookie cutter and finely cut out circles

6. Put the processed dough into the pan and pre-heat your oven to a temperature of 325 degree Fahrenheit

7. Prepare all of the ingredients- mince up your garlic, chop up your onions and slice your mushroom

8. Gently Sauté your onion and garlic by tossing them in olive oil

9. Once done, toss in the ground beef and sear them finely

10. Pour in the Worcestershire and Spices

11. Then, toss in the mushrooms and mix them all as well

12. Add in the tomato paste and enough mustard before finishing it up

13. Gently, spoon the ground beef mixture and push them in your pastry tartlets and cover them up with cheese.

14. Finally, bake them for about 20-25 minutes

15. Cool it and eat

Nutrition Values(Total)

- Protein: 144g
- Carbs: 49.3g
- Fats: 213g
- Calories: 2648
- Fiber: 19.2g

A Very Private and Intimate Portobello Pizza

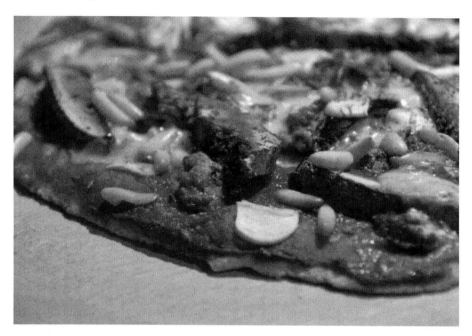

Serving And Preparation Time

The following recipe is going to yield 4 serving and will take about 15 minutes to make and prepare.

Ingredients

For the Bun

- 4 pieces of large sized Portobello Mushroom Caps

- 1 medium sized Vine Tomato

- 4 ounce of Fresh Mozzarella Cheese

- ¼ cup of Freshly Chopped up Basil

- 6 tablespoon of Olive Oil

- 20 slices of Pepperoni

- Salt as needed

- Pepper as needed

How To

1. Take your mushroom and scrape out the internals until just a shell remains

2. Turn over the shells and broil them

3. Coat the top with about 3 tablespoon of olive oil

4. Season with pepper and salt upon rubbing with the oil

5. Broil the mushrooms for 5 minutes making sure to flip them up

6. Slice your tomato into thin slices and lay them on top of your mushroom alongside fresh basil

7. Place your Pepperoni and cubed cheese on top of each mushroom and broil once more for 4 minutes (making sure that the cheese is molten and slightly brown)

8. Take it out and serve

Nutrition Values(Per Serving)

- Protein: 8.5g

- Carbs: 4g

- Fats: 31g

- Calories: 320

- Fiber: 1.25g

Egg Drop Soup Of 5 Minutes

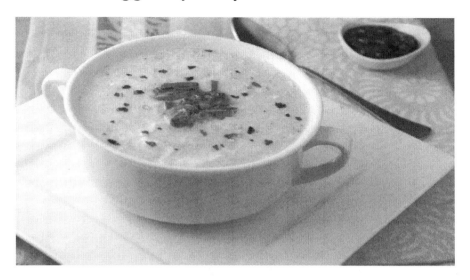

Serving And Preparation Time

The following recipe is going to yield 1 serving and will take about 6 minutes to make and prepare.

Ingredients

- 1 and a ½ cup of chicken broth
- ½ a cube of Chicken Bouillon
- 1 tablespoon of butter
- 2 large sized eggs
- 1 teaspoon of Chili Garlic Paste

How To

1. Take your pan and put it on top of a stove and turn it to medium-high heat
2. Toss in the chicken broth, bacon fat, bouillon cube into the pan

3. Once the broth has come to a boil, toss in the garlic paste and keep stirring it. Then turn off your stove

4. Take a bowl and beat up your eggs and pour the mixture into the steaming broth

5. Keep stirring it and finally let it sit for a while before serving.

Nutrition Values (Per Serving)

- Protein: 12g

- Carbs: 2.5g

- Fats: 23g

- Calories: 276

Amazing Raspberry Pavlovas

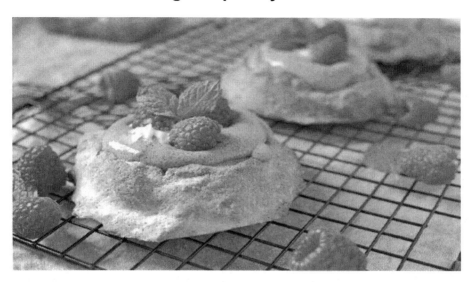

Serving And Preparation Time

The following recipe is going to yield 6 serving and will take about 10 minutes to make and prepare.

Ingredients

For the Base

- 4 pieces of large egg whites
- ½ a cup of Erythritol
- 1 teaspoon of Vanilla Extract
- 1 teaspoon of Fresh lemon Juice
- 2 teaspoon of Xanthan Gum

For the Filling

- 1 cup of Heavy Cream
- 85g of Frozen Berries

For the topping

- 18 pieces of Fresh Raspberries
- 1-2 pieces of Min Leaves

How To

1. Pre-heat you oven to a temperature of 300 Degree Fahrenheit
2. Separate 4 eggs and carefully them white out of them until a foamy texture appears
3. Toss in the Erythritol drop by drop while beating it
4. Keep mixing it until stiff peaks
5. Pour in the vanilla, xanthan gum and lemon juice
6. Fold the mixture using a silicone spatula
7. Line up a baking sheet using a parchment paper and take a pencil to outline the cup to be used as a guideline for your pavlova mixture
8. Spoon up the pavlova batter and place in the drawn circle
9. Bake them for about 60 minutes
10. On the side, prepare the filling by measuring out 85g of frozen berries
11. Blend them with a cup of heavy cream for 3 minutes and scoop them up
12. Place the scooped up berries in your pavlova and serve

Nutrition Values (Per Serving)

- Protein: 3.2g
- Carbs: 4g
- Fats: 15g
- Calories: 162

Magical Cashew Bars (No Bake Required)

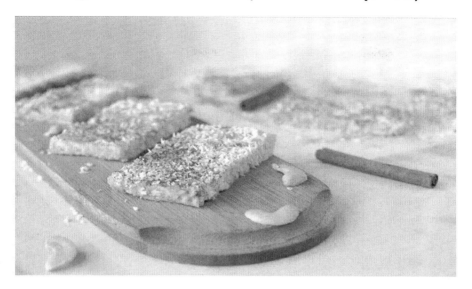

Serving And Preparation Time

The following recipe is going to yield 8 serving and will take about 2 hours to make and prepare.

Ingredients

- 1 cup of Almond Flour
- ¼ cup of butter
- ¼ cup of Sugar Free Maple Syrup
- 1 teaspoon of Cinnamon
- 1 pinch of Salt
- ½ a cup of Cashew Nut
- ¼ cup of shredded Coconut

How To

1. Combine the molten butter alongside the almond flour using a large bowl

2. Toss in the salt, cinnamon, shredded coconut and pour the maple syrup to mix them well

3. Roughly chop up about ½ a cup of cashew nuts and add them to your mixture

4. Take a baking dish lined with parchment paper and spread out the dough evenly in a layer

5. Freeze it for about 2 hours and then serve by cutting them into bars

Nutrition Values(Per Serving)

- Protein: 4.4g

- Carbs: 6.1g

- Fats: 17g

- Calories: 189

Mesmerizing Lemon Soufflé!

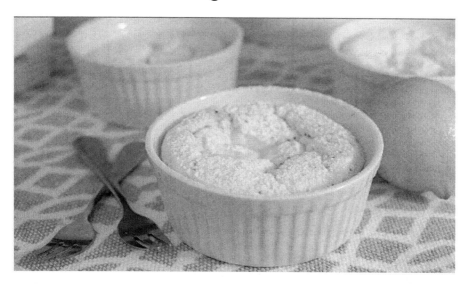

Serving And Preparation Time

The following recipe is going to yield 1 serving and will take about 25 minutes to make and prepare.

Ingredients

- 1 cup of Whole Milk Ricotta
- 2 separated Large sized Eggs
- ¼ cup of Erythritol
- 2 teaspoon of Lemon Zest
- 1 tablespoon of Fresh Lemon Juice
- 1 teaspoon of Vanilla Extract
- 1 teaspoon of Poppy Seeds

How To

1. Pre-heat your oven to a temperature of 375 degree Fahrenheit

2. Take two bowls and separate 2 eggs into the bowls

3. Beat them until foamy

4. Pour in about 2 tablespoon of Erythritol and beat them finely

5. In another bowl, toss in the ricotta cheese, egg yolk and 2 tablespoon of Erythritol

6. Into the creamy mixture, pour in the half of a lemon juice and zest

7. Pour in the vanilla extract and toss the poppy seeds as well

8. Mix them up and fold the egg yolks half at one time, stirring it very gently

9. Take 4 ramekins and grease them up and pour your batter into them

10. Shake it up to flatten out the top

11. Bake for 20 minutes and serve

Nutrition Values

- Protein: 9g
- Carbs: 3g
- Fats: 10g
- Calories: 151

Conclusion

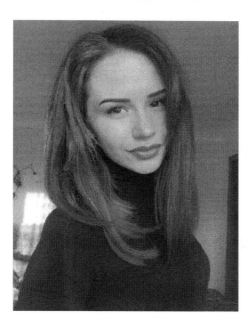

I would like to thank you for purchasing and downloading my book. I really do hope that you had a pleasant time with my book and enjoyed reading it.

I bid you farewell and hope that your Keto journey may turn out to be a huge success! I would feel that I have accomplished my mission even I had a tiny contribution into helping you achieve a healthy lifestyle

Stay healthy and stay safe.

Made in the USA
Lexington, KY
27 January 2018